FOOD, SWEAT, & FEARS

Denise
(my Tiny Wool Spule)
thank you for everything.

God Bless

REGINA BARTLETT

ISBN: 9781980555384

DEDICATION

This book is dedicated to the most important people in my life.

My husband Jeff Bartlett for his unwavering love and support throughout our lives together. Jeff, thank you for always supporting me, believing in me, and loving me – especially when it was particularly hard for me to love myself.

My parents Richard & Ramona Foster for going above and beyond for the wellbeing of my children and myself through some of the toughest times of my life. There are few things as precious as the unconditional love of parents and children. I will work tirelessly every day to make sure you know how much I appreciate you for all you have done and sacrificed for Darienne, Nicholas, and me.

REGINA BARTLETT

BEFORE YOU BEGIN

Thank you for taking the time to read *Food, Sweat, & Fears*. This is not a traditional book by any means. It's a series of events through my life with regard to my weight loss and my journey with Christ through running the NYC Marathon. It's not – nor was it meant to be – a complete memoir or even in sequential order. Each chapter handles a certain aspect of my life but there are many details that aren't directly related to the main themes of this book and are left out. Every event here is real but many of the names have been changed or deliberately left out. As you read consider it a peek into a diary of events. If you've been following my writing over the course of the past decade then some of these chapters may sound familiar. They are expanded version of blogs that I have written in the past and were germane to this story.

Thank you again for your support.

God Bless!

Regina Bartlett

CONTENTS

Acknowledgments iii

1 New Year's Day 2014 1

2 A History of Failure 5

3 A Bitter Divorce 19

4 Regina Runs 33

5 Introducing Love & Mopeds 55

6 Shedding For The Wedding 70

7 Introducing Another Love 85

8 Another Day Another Diet 96

9 Visually Disturbing 103

i

10 My Guilty Valentine   106

11 Food Funerals   116

12 Surgery Day & Too Much Time   131

13 Hot and Ready Car Ride   143

14 Elbowing In The Kitchen   150

15 The Beauty of Being Seen   157

16 The Summer of Living   166

17 The Longest Marathon   177

18 The Five "F" Words   201

19 Final Word   214

ACKNOWLEDGMENTS

All glory to Jesus! The depth of His love for me has opened up every possible joy in my life. Acknowledging His all-encompassing love has enabled me to see love in all people and all situations and in myself…which was often the hardest place to love. RFB

John 3:16

CHAPTER ONE
NEW YEAR'S DAY 2014

In an instant my knee exploded in pain. I grabbed onto the handrail and felt it give from the wall. If I fall down these stairs, it's over. Drywall powder came out of the wall where the screw was coming out but then settled. I was still upright. Thank you, Jesus. I don't know what would've happened if I fell. Falling down stairs is bad enough but at my size it can be fatal. The last thing I want is for my daughter who is home on Christmas break from college to find me hurt or worse when she wakes up.

I got my balance and managed to set myself down on the stairs. This was the third time this week that my knee has gone out. It feels like the kneecap is trying to escape.

Climbing the stairs is getting harder every day. I know I'm over 400lbs again. When I hit 400lbs basic movement becomes a challenge. I know I'm there.

Just then my daughter bounded out of the room. She thought she heard something and saw me on the stairs.

"Are you ok?" she asked clearly concerned.

"Yes, I'm fine," I lie. I'm absolutely not fine.

"Ok good, let's go clean your office. It's the new year! It's time to get rid of the old and greet the new," she exclaims with too much vigor this early in the morning.

I continued up the stairs hiding the pain from her as we walked into the office. My heart is beating out of my chest. Half a flight of steps and I'm immediately out of breath.

We start purging the office and she is relentless. It's always my nature to want to keep things that I may need in the future. She wants to throw absolutely everything away. She uses the logic that you can always get it again. Is she my child? She definitely takes after her grandmother. Every few minutes I have to sit down but the doesn't let me. For hours we work and clean and organize. Any moment the warden isn't looking I try to take a seat. My breath is heaving from my chest and I'm thinking of what I could possibly give her that she will love enough to let me rest. There is nothing, we continue to work.

When it was done my office was beautiful. A place for everything and everything in its place. I plunked down on the futon in the corner of my office and took a break.

"Mom, give me your phone. I want to send some pictures to grandma, she's going to be so proud of you," she said with a sense of pride in her voice.

I gave her my phone without even opening my eyes. I could hear her snapping away as I fell asleep.

A few hours later I decided to take a look at those pictures and as I scrolled I was pretty proud of myself. Look at that organization. Maybe this is the year of living organized! In the midst of my joy I saw something that took my breath away. I was never so embarrassed. I immediately went to the text messages to see if she sent this pic to my mother. She did. I felt the color drain from my face.

There I was lying on the futon with my headscarf on and my body took up the entire futon. This photo showed absolutely everything I ever wanted to hide in a picture. It showed how tired I look, how sad I looked, and how my weight has claimed me. I was defeated.

Once you see something you can't unsee it. That picture stayed in the back of my mind forever. I couldn't let it go. I also couldn't 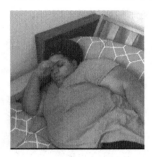 delete it. Sometimes, I'd stare at it and berate myself for continuing to fail.

Why am I so overweight?

Why can't I keep to a diet?

Why do I try and fail over and over again?

What's it going to take to be successful?

CHAPTER TWO

A HISTORY OF FAILURE

I remember clearly the day my weight became an issue. I was 12 years old and going to the clinic for a physical for school. The nurse escorted me to the scale and I stepped on it. Didn't seem like a big deal at all. Little did I know it was the beginning of what would become the most anxious time of my life.

As soon as I stepped on the scale the weight bar hit like a brick on the other side. She moved the weight bar further down and it teetered then finally balanced. The scale read about 150lbs. She then scrawled some notes on the chart and gave it to me to bring into the room for the doctor. As soon as I walked in the exam room I looked at the chart to see what she wrote. There it was in print:

Grossly Overweight.

Not just overweight.

Not chubby.

Grossly overweight.

Even at 12 years old I knew that I had steadily gained weight. I knew it the day my mother brought home Husky pants for school. I knew it when FAT was the first thing a kid will say to insult me on the playground. I knew it. Now, it seemed like everyone knew it and my doctor was about to know it as well.

I could feel the pit in my stomach. As I sat in the office I was quickly thinking of what to say if he asks me about my weight. What could I tell him? The truth?

The truth was that I never liked uncomfortable things. I come from a large family where I bring up the rear as the sixth of seven children. My siblings are all very athletic and outgoing and funny. I was always different. I was quieter than most and not much of an athlete. A good day to me was reading everything I could get my hands on. When all the kids wanted to go outside and play I was perfectly content with a book in my room. My exploration always occurred inwardly.

Being different was something I tended to notice about myself, not exactly what others thought of me. I kept judging myself against the standards of my family and friends. I was always really hard on myself. Putting so much pressure on myself was a lot to handle. When faced with discomfort, you seek comfort. I discovered comfort in food.

As much as I don't remember the day that food became important to me I do remember what I started doing. I would steal cookies from the cupboard and eat them in my room. When that became too noticeable I would take entire packages of cookies right after my mom came back from shopping. It was less noticeable to take a whole carton then to take most of them out.

I'll never forget the day I got caught. My mother decided to clean my room and she discovered several empty packages of cookies. She put everything in a pile and when I opened the door I thought I was going to pass out. I was caught! She left a note on the pile that said she wanted it clean before she came home, and she never wanted to see the wrappers in my room again. I cleaned my room and we never mentioned the wrappers again.

I wish I could say that I never stole food from the pantry after that, but I absolutely did. I just got better about disposing of evidence. I'd throw out the contents of old board games that we rarely played and I would hide food wrappers in the box. Every time someone would want to play a board game I'd hold my breath and pray that they didn't pick Life or Parcheesi again. It never looked like I was eating very much but I was continuing to gain weight.

I was NOT about to share this with the doctor. I decided that if he said anything at all I would just agree with whatever he said to do and be done with it.

Waiting for him to enter was nerve wracking. I just wanted to go home. What is he going to say? What am I going to have to do? What if he tells my parents? What if they put me on a diet? The questions rolled through my brain one after the other and I was freaking myself out. By the time he entered I was ready for the worst. He probably saw the look of worried desperation on my face and said: *Try to lose a few pounds before your physical next year.*

WHAT?

THAT'S IT?

I was almost disappointed that was all he said. In the ten minutes I was waiting for him I convinced myself he was going to ship me off to Fat Camp! I left the office shaking but ready to explore what I can do to lose weight.

I got home and turned on the television. The commercial for Richard Simmons's Deal a Meal was on and I was enthralled. I was fascinated by Richard Simmons. I loved his larger than life personality and how he genuinely seemed to care for the people on his shows and in his videos.

Deal A Meal looked amazing and simple to follow. It was a little plastic holder that had a set of cards that contained certain food groups. Depending on what you needed to lose and the calorie requirements for your size you put those specific cards on the left. As soon as you ate something from the card you moved it from the left to the right. When all of your cards were on the right you were done with food for the day. Simple! I knew that this could be the answer. I just need to shift cards as I ate. That would surely allow me to lose weight. I went to my parents and I begged to order a Deal A Meal kit. They weren't as impressed with Richard Simmons as I was, and they turned me down.

Over the next few weeks my eating habits didn't change at all and I was still gaining weight. People were starting to pick on me more and more for my size and it was getting harder to be grossly overweight. I wanted to change my habits and I just knew that Deal A Meal was the answer.

I went to my parents again asked them to really look at how many people Richard Simmons has helped over the years and just imagine that I could be one of them. I offered up my meager wages from babysitting to help with the purchase. I think they saw how serious I was because they relented and paid for Deal A Meal. I even got to keep my babysitting money. I waited for weeks for the box to arrive. Back in the day, we actually had to wait longer than 48 hours for something you ordered to come in the mail. When I opened the box, it was like my new life was sitting inside. I was ready.

The first few days were amazing. I learned a lot about food and food groups. I was very good at moving my cards over and I was losing weight. It was amazing. Richard

Simmons became a god to me. Look at what he's able to do. What a genius program.

After a couple of weeks, I was really starting to miss cookies. I decided that I could make some accommodations on the cards. If I could have a sandwich on my cards, I'd have two cookies instead of two slices of bread. It's about the same, right? Sure, it is.

Then I started not moving the cards every time I ate. I'd just hold a couple of cards back and use them later. Did Richard know that his system was inherently flawed? It became very easy to game the Deal A Meal system. Before long any progress I made was lost. Clearly it was Richard Simmons' fault.

My weight continued to rise throughout Junior High and High School. By my early twenties I was well over 200lbs. With every passing year, every poor relationship, and every stressful job food became my method of handling anything.

Pain? Food.

Fear? Food.

Challenges? Food.

Joy? Food.

Celebration? Food.

Birthday? Definitely food.

Flash forward 15 years after Deal A Meal and I'm a single mother of two kids, balancing a crazy work situation, and struggling constantly. Food was the answer to every single question. My weight was going to kill me but I couldn't stop eating.

By my early thirties I started getting chest tightness. Being overweight, constantly stressed, and generally not taking care of myself I knew I had to do something. My father's mother died at a very young age from a heart attack and we shared the same body type. The chest pains were scaring me. I had to go to the doctor.

Going to the doctor as a heavy person is traumatic. You almost never want to say that something is wrong because the only answer is to lose weight. Any symptom is just reflective of your weight problem. I'm already anxious that I'm in the office and I know that I'll have to get on the scale. It had been years since I weighed myself.

The nurse walks me over to the scale. She takes a look at me and changes the weights.

She starts me at the 250. I immediately have a flashback to my 12-year-old grossly overweight self and I proceed to take off anything that wouldn't be perceived as indecent to remove. Earrings, glasses, shoes, change from my pockets, keys. I go step on and for a second think if it would be weird if I took off my socks. Then I remembered that 100 people have probably stepped on that that scale today, so the socks stayed on and I got on.

The sound of the bar slamming down was alarming. I'm apparently over 250lbs. She moved the slide weight slowly at first, but the lever didn't move at all. She slapped it all the way to the end. The lever didn't even budge. She picked up the larger weight and put it on the 300 and the slide weight is still at the far end. I'm not quick on the math in my head but I knew that this was not good. Her eyes open pretty wide and she caught herself then looked at me with absolute pity.

"I can't get your weight on this scale. I'm sorry," she said.

"How much is that?" I ask.

"It stops at 350lbs." She averted her eyes and I stepped down.

Humiliated. Demoralized. She escorts me to the exam room and as soon as the door closes I begin to cry wondering if there is any possible way I could feel worse than I did at that moment.

After sitting in my misery for about 20 minutes the doctor entered.

'Well, how are you, Regina?" He's looking over my chart.

"I'm okay, I guess. I've been having some odd pains that are starting to concern me."

"What concerns me is that we can't get your weight in the office," he is still looking at my chart.

"Is there another place to get my weight?"

"I'd suggest making an appointment at the main post office in Providence. They have a freight scale and can get your accurate weight." He never even looked up from his chart.

The freight scale. I thought not being able to be weighed would be the lowest I could possibly feel. Hearing the weight slam on the scale was like the undertow but the freight scale suggestion was definitely taking me under. I don't remember the rest of the appointment. I just vowed that I would never be in this position again. I needed to do something.

I started with starvation. Excellent place to start. I convinced myself that the secret to success lies in not eating any food at all. I can do it. Just water and air, that's all I really needed. I could live off my body fat for years. So, I set about my new starvation diet. How hard could it be?

By noon of Day One I realized that not eating anything wasn't going to happen. I had to do something else. While I sat and thought about what means of dieting I could try I ate some cookies. This was going to be harder than I thought. After much deliberation and several snacks, I decided that I would just try to eat more responsibly and see how that goes.

It didn't go at all. It seemed like the more I tried not to focus on what I was eating I would eat out of control but coincidentally the more I focused on what I was eating all I wanted to do was eat. How was I ever going to combat this?

This struggled continued for years. I would put forth some effort, take strides, and within no time at all return to exactly where I was but worse. I noticed that when my weight was better I felt better, and I did more outgoing things. When my weight was decidedly off the rails I isolated myself and tended to avoid my issues both personally and financially.

As my weight climbed I also began to struggle more with social anxiety although I didn't know what that was at the time. I just knew that there were times when the thought of answering a phone call would send panic through me. I didn't know why but it was beginning to wreak havoc on my life. I needed more control over this, but I feared that I would never have it. I thought about seeing a therapist, but I had flashbacks to my first and only therapy session.

Winter 2003. I sat uncomfortably in the chair staring at the doctor staring across from me. I'm initially distracted because I thought I'd be stretched on a couch and comfortable. Instead I'm in a staring contest with Dr. Silence who has not said a single word since I entered his office. After our moment of silence, he asked me two questions.

"So, Regina, do you have a boyfriend?"

"No," I answered totally shocked that he decided to go there first.

"What about your weight, are you happy with your weight?"

"No," I answered again this time for shocked than the last time.

He took out a prescription pad and starting scrawling quickly. He looked at me and said, "Take this and I'll see you next week."

As I walked out I wondered what just happened? That was therapy? Based solely on television sitcoms I had a completely different view of what therapy would be like and that wasn't it. So, based on this doctor's logic if I had a boyfriend or wasn't fat I'd have no issues whatsoever. I was trying not to have a bad attitude about it despite how I felt leaving the office.

I picked up the prescription and stared at it for a while. I wasn't sure what to expect but I took it anyway and since it was my day off I felt it was the best day to try something new. For the first hour I didn't feel any differently but slowly but surely, I started to feel the effects. It was like everything was moving slowly and I wasn't reacting the same. There was a profound sense of calm that in the next hour felt more like I was drifting into a coma.

So much for that experiment. There was no way I was taking anything that took me so far out of myself. I was supposed to try the prescribed dosage and then report back to the doctor with how I was feeling. I felt like the doctor was a waste of my time and I never returned.

It's more than a decade after that therapeutic ordeal and I'm no better than I was before. Still no boyfriend, still not happy about my weight, but now I leave the doctor's office wondering if I would ever have the strength to contact the Post Office to make an appointment to get weighed. No, I won't do that.

Instead, I left and got a bag of Oreos and ate every single one before I even got home.

CHAPTER THREE

A BITTER DIVORCE

Food was my sole source of comfort for a long time. As my weight continued to grow I stumbled upon something quite by accident that changed my eating habits but gave me another different habit.

I was at a house party in 1989, and we were all having a blast. Looking back now we must have looked a sight with our side ponytails, multiple pairs of socks, and enough hair spray to launch a rocket to the moon. Everyone was getting along just fine and then out of nowhere a fight broke out. It was instant pandemonium.

One guy brought his new younger girlfriend to the party and his ex-girlfriend wasn't too thrilled about her being there. Insults were flying, and everyone was trying to diffuse the situation which only managed to make it worse. I left the backyard and went to sit on the front porch. To this day I don't remember who was there but they had a pack of menthol Benson & Hedges cigarettes and the mystery person offered me one.

I remember that first cigarette well. Most people have stories about how their first cigarette was the worst experience of their lives. For me, it felt like home. I never coughed or choked, and it was smooth and easy. I liked it right away.

Rhode Island increased the age to purchase cigarettes from 16 to 18 in 1988, but they were surprisingly easy to come by in 1989. Our school even had a smoking section! Smoking was frowned upon but not like today and a lot of parents smoked so getting cigarettes was a breeze. It wasn't long before I was buying them myself, but it was never going to be a long-term thing. I did notice that as long as I smoked I wasn't eating so that was a good side benefit for cigarettes.

After a few months I decided my smoke of choice was Marlboro Red 100s. I was paying about $1.90 for a pack of cigarettes which was more than the cost of a gallon of gas. I was just going to smoke for a few months and be done. Again, not a long-term thing. I decided that no matter what I will stop smoking when cigarettes cost more than $2 a pack. That was an insane price for a pack of anything so there was no way I was going to pay $2 for a pack of smokes! No way! NEVER!

It was hot day in the summer of 1990, and I'm in a rush on my way to work. There was no way I was going to survive another shift working in retail at the beach without a pack of cigarettes. I stop at a gas station and I take out two crispy dollar bills and run into the store.

"Pack of Marlboro Red 100s, please." I say.

"That's $2.05," he says.

It felt like I was hit with a pound of bricks to the face. WHAT? Seriously?

"I just brought in $2.00," thinking he may let me slide.

"Then perhaps you should go back out," he replies as he pulls the pack back from my reach.

I swore that I would quit the minute cigarettes cost over $2 per pack. I was also quite confident that day would not come around so quickly. I was at a crossroads. I took my two dollars and went back to my car. I calmly got a nickel from my console and proceed to get my cigarettes. This was just the first of many promises I would break to myself and others about smoking.

College took my smoking to a whole new level. Staying up at all hours of the night to finish a paper and then sprint across the quad to turn it in while it was still hot from the printer. Those nights were made possible not by copious amounts of caffeine and cigarettes. I mastered the art of one handed typing so that I could smoke and continue to write.

When I was pregnant in early 1994, I left my doctor's appointment and took my pack of smokes and tossed them out the window. I was in this for the greater good. And I did it. I was smoke free and with a new baby smoking was the furthest thing from my mind.

When I went back to work, I discovered that I was programmed to smoke. You know when you are on an elevator and the bell rings and the door opens, and you just start to get out? You don't look to see if it's your floor you just go. Why? Because we are exactly as

Pavlov discovered, we are programmed. Elevator bell rings, door opens, you leave. I would work for a few hours, take a break, and go outside to smoke. Programmed.

Smoking at work also had social implications. The smoking section is where we gathered, shared news, talked shop, got the low down on everything happening at work at beyond. It was our version of the water cooler. Who was going to miss that social time? Clearly, not me.

I really think I only liked smoking for about the first 6 months then I couldn't stand it. The expense was one thing but the fact that you're tied to this beast that made your clothing smell was just crazy to continue. But I earnestly continued.

I have rarely smoked in front of my children. I was definitely an outdoor and late-night smoker for the most part. But they knew I smoked and always asked me to quit. I made multiple promises to try.

This brings us to 2007, in our local Walmart. I had just purchased a condo and we had a lot of household stuff to get. The kids and I were going through the aisles getting the "stuff."

My daughter needed face wash which was near the pharmacy. She selects a $10

Neutrogena Acne Wash and I nearly pass out. Ten bucks? Then I think of all the possibilities of teenage skin and decide it's worth its weight in gold.

We walk past the pharmacy and she stops. She goes directly to the Smoking Cessation Center, yes, Smoking Cessation Center and picks up "the Patch."

I give her a look. She returns the look. We are now locked in an epic stare down over the Nicoderm box in the Walmart Pharmacy.

"Oh, I don't need that! I'm going to quit," I say.

"You always say that, but you never do," she replied. No fear or retreat with this one.

"I will, I just need some more time."

"You are going to run out of time!" Her voice is raising and my attitude is too.

"That is enough young lady," I'm actively trying convey how I'm not going to hear too much more of this.

"No, Mom, get it today. You promised!"

I decide not to say a single word. I was just going to stare at her until she could feel that I am no longer playing this game with her in the store. Then she said something that disarmed me completely. I wasn't ready for it at all.

"You gave me my life and now I am saving yours!"

She had a fire in her eyes that I had never seen and as much as I was trying to communicate that I was done with this conversation, she communicated even more how she was the one not taking any more of my baloney. There was only one thing left to do. I asked the pharmacist for a box of the patch. I paid $41 for a two week supply of Nicoderm. That was almost the cost of smoking!

The following morning before I went to work I placed the patch on my arm and went out the door. I feared my Pavlov programmed mind would tempt me to smoke on my break but then the fear of potentially dying from smoking a cigarette while wearing the patch seemed to take that away.

I was warned by many people that you can get really vivid nightmares while using the patch. Quite the opposite happened to me. I rarely ever remember my dreams but the two weeks I had on the patch gave me vivid and amazing dreams. It was like a new adventure every night.

After the first week, I had a good routine going.

1. Wake up
2. Take a shower
3. Dry off
4. Locate yet another patch of skin to place the patch
5. Get dressed
6. Notice the patch is on my clothes, not my skin
7. Remove patch from blouse
8. Re-press on skin
9. Move one inch
10. Repeat steps 7-9 for next 16 waking hours

The hardest part was step 4. I didn't think that finding a new skin location would be the hardest thing I would do all day, but it really was. You can't just slap it anywhere and move on. The location has to be free of hair. Fair enough, who wants a nicotine sticker on a patch of hair? And isn't this common sense? But I would like to know what happened to the person that called to complain that it ripped all their arm hair so that the disclaimer is on the box! There is always one!

The location also cannot sweat. Now this can sometimes be challenging since was April in Providence where one day it's hot and the next freezing. The indoor temperature varies about 40 degrees an hour just trying to keep up with what is going on outside. All New Englanders are sick during early spring because of this temperature variance. It all add to the challenge to find a bald patch of sweat less skin.

Once you find a good spot you have the additional struggle of trying to remove the patch. I would spend 15 minutes in the shower just trying to remove the nico-glue from my skin only to go to work and have it surface there again.. I would do it again. It would come back. You know that grass that comes out only at Easter to put in the kids' baskets? You clean it up and 6 months later you find it again in some random spot like you never cleaned it at all? It's like that. Rings of nico-glue everywhere. Then I discovered Baby Oil. Easy, fast, and clean. Miracle Oil.

Working on the patch was definitely an adventure. For the most part people are very supportive. Most people. Then there are those that will just tell you outright that they will see you in the smoking section very soon. Thanks, you are so kind.

I managed to keep my Pavlovian instincts at bay when everyone was going out to smoke. I even survived a real test of strength: Boredom. It was raining outside and not much going on inside. I watched a little TV, surfed a little of the internet, had a little dinner, and was getting a little bored. I really could have done it that night. Smoking would have been just what filled that space. I thought about it long and hard. I could smoke just ONE. It was tempting. The thought was almost beautiful. Then I realized one essential truth:

I could NEVER just smoke one cigarette.

I decided to be strong, let the craving pass, and just have a little faith in myself!

Two weeks after quitting my cousin Sybil was diagnosed with lung cancer. Sybil was an amazing woman. She was smart, funny, tall with a gorgeous smile, two beautiful boys and a wonderful husband that she had been with since college. She and her sister were so close they were like the dynamic duo and as my older cousins they were always people I looked up to. When Sybil was diagnosed with lung cancer she handled it like everything else in her life: head on and with passion.

She never smoked a day. As much as I was struggling to keep myself from smoking her diagnosis really put my efforts into overdrive. It wasn't fair that I was a smoker and she was the one with cancer! I had a renewed sense of willpower and a desire to do this for her.

My surprise with quitting smoking was not that I wanted to smoke but that my hands really wanted something to do. I smoked a lot so my hands were always occupied. I found a book on origami and started to learn the beautiful Japanese art of paper folding. I started with cubes and stars and then Then a diamond. A bat. A cup. The three dimensional items really took me away. I found something to do with my hands that doesn't involve a lighter or slowly killing myself. Eureka!

Then it started doing it all the time. Making boxes after boxes, diamonds, animals. I was obsessed. I liked the challenge of it. When I got really comfortable with the 3D objects I was making I decided to see if I could make them smaller. I went to smaller sheets of origami paper. It was a breeze. So I went smaller. And smaller. I thought it was an accomplishment to make a box out of a Post-It. The gummy edge posed a challenge that I relished.

You would think that someone who successfully make an origami 3D box with a Post-It would take a moment and really breathe in that victory. NOPE. I embarked upon the ultimate challenge. I looked at it for a second. I tried to be sure that I was ready for it. I did the math in my head a thousand times. I knew it could be done I just had to believe. Then I did it. I made the box. I made the box out of a **Starburst candy wrapper**. It was beautiful.

All of this paper folding made me see exactly what I was really doing when I was smoking. I fell on smoking for everything. I needed a breather? Smoking. I needed to think? Smoking. I was hungry? Smoking. Bored? Smoking! I thought I would never find something that I could do that would take that away.

After a few months I drove everyone I knew crazy with the origami. I had a house full of boxes, stars, and cranes. I decided to channel this craziness into a project. Remembering the book *Sadako and the Thousand Paper Cranes* that my kids read in school, I embarked on a mission to make 1000 cranes to send to Japan for the International Day of Peace in August.

When my sister in law saw the cranes she asked me if she could put her name on one. I thought that was a great idea so I wrote her name on the neck of the crane. I was a Myspace blogger with a decent amount of readers and decided to reach out to them to see if anyone also wanted a name on a crane.

The response was overwhelming. I needed 999 names and I thought I may get about 500. Within hours I had over 1200 names and I didn't want to commit to anymore since I still had to fold them all.

By the end of July 2007, I had completed 1200 cranes roped in a groups of 100 and sent them off to Japan. I didn't have to make them all because some of my friends and family pitched in and helped. It was amazing and a huge sense of accomplishment.

After 18 years I was finally smoke free and just completed a project that really changed my life. Things were looking great. I was so optimistic. Then we got the call that Sybil had passed away. She fought fiercely and was laid to rest in August 2007. We were all devastated.

Tomorrow is guaranteed to no one.

I successfully divorced smoking but rekindled my previous affair with food with reckless abandon. By early 2008, I had gained well over 100lbs by eating my grief and guilt and not having cigarettes to temper the cravings.

CHAPTER FOUR
REGINA RUNS

After I quit smoking and before my crazy obsession with origami I had another venture. In early 2007, I transferred jobs in the same company to the corporate office in the city. The building was beautiful and we had a nicely equipped gym in the basement. I joined the gym at my first location and my membership transferred to this new location. As an employee only gym it was pennies a day to join and it was automatically deducted from my paycheck.

I did have the opportunity to experience both gyms and from what I have seen most of the employees in both buildings pay for a membership but only a fraction actually use them. They could be considered "vanity memberships." A vanity membership is when you decide that you want to join a gym hoping that you might actually go. Thinking that you may actually show up because you are paying for it.

Employee Gym By The Numbers
Number of people in building: 800
Number of gym memberships: 225
Number of people who actually go: 110
Number of times I went at my old location: 5
Number of times at my new location: 0

In April I went to see the gym where I had my vanity-transferred-membership and I saw a sign advertising a charity 5k that is run in different locations all over the world. I wanted to become a real member not a vanity member so I asked about the 5k. I had 2 months to train.

The race supplied our corporate team with training information to take you from the couch to running a 5k. The couch I could handle, the 5K Training wasn't easy. I would go walking but not long enough and not often enough. I had every excuse as to why I couldn't possibly train. Race day was approaching and I was concerned.

I thought about just bailing on the race but there were some caveats. I already paid for the race, I designed the shirts for my company and EVERYONE knows I'm supposed to be there since I all but harassed everyone to doing it with me.

I tried to convince myself that it's only 3.2 miles and how bad could it be?

June 28, 2007.
Race Day. Boston.
15,000 participants.
Everyone is there.
Press.
Sponsors.
Announcers.
Serious Runners.
Regina.

Fresh off of very little sleep wearing the t-shirt that I designed walking to the start with over 75 others from my company looking like a solid mass of bright red that didn't want to be messed with. Have you ever seen 15,000 people outside of a concert? That is what the starting gate looked like. Just a sea of people. The starting gate is right in front of us. I look to my right the sign reads:

5MIN/MILE   START HERE

I couldn't run a 5 minute mile unless I was being chased by someone with a gun. Another one of my co-workers was also run challenged and decided we needed to get out of that area or we'd get trampled at the start. It isn't easy to get through that many people so we stopped at this sign:

10MIN/MILE   START HERE

The announcer yells "Runners, take your mark!"

I'm thinking: "What about brisk walkers?"

And then BAM! The gun goes off and all of the 10,000 people behind me take off like a shot. I couldn't imagine if I had stayed in the 5min/mile area. I paced a jog and we were so far back we had gone a literally a half a mile BEFORE we even got to the gate. Then something amazing happened. In that glorious sea of human beings each with their own reasons for being there I found why I was there.

I have the soul of a runner.

I loved the feeling of freedom I had out there. I loved the way I felt. Whatever tension I had disappearing the further I went. Just when I was ready to really melt into this running thing. I got a little more focused. I alternated between jogging and walking but even when I walked I wanted to keep a decent pace. I did just that and I did it until the end.

When I saw the finish line I thought I was going to cry. Not from pain but from accomplishment. I wasn't concerned with the official time. I was in a completely different place: I said I would do it and I did. What else could I do?

I decided to register for more races. I signed up for a couple of 5ks and a Half Marathon! The Half Marathon wasn't until February so I had plenty of time to train. I could do this.

I found myself outside at all hours and discovered how clear my mind is when I'm out there. It became easier to keep a steady jog after a while. I was improving. My next race was the morning of my 35th birthday and I couldn't wait.

September 7, 2007, was the night before my birthday 5k. Living in the city it wasn't necessary to drive and I couldn't afford a car anyway. The race was in North Kingstown, RI, which is in the suburbs so I was checking the bus schedule because the busses go there, not too often, but they do go there. I wanted to make sure everything went off without a hitch.

The bus map on the bus schedule only provides times for major cross streets and landmarks. Google Maps gives everything down to number of shrubs in someone's yard. I would take the bus listed cross streets and Google Map it to find out how far away I would have to walk to get to the school. After what seemed like an eternity I found one that was about a mile away. Seemed like a perfect warm up for the 5k!

The race was scheduled to start at 9:30AM so to get from my house to the connecting bus I had to leave at 6:30AM to catch the 7:30AM bus to the 'burbs. I would have some time to wait but I figured it would be good to get me up and keep me awake. I made sure the iPod was charged and everything was laid out. It was going to be great!

I woke up without incident and I was at my bus stop with plenty of time to spare. The connecting bus arrived on time and asked the driver if he could get me as close to the high school as possible. He asked me where it was. I knew right there I was in trouble. I gave him my Google Map cross streets. He had no idea where they were. He pretty much pulls the bus over if one of three things happen:

- ➤ Someone pulls the cord. He will stop at next stop marked with a blue bus.
- ➤ Someone is standing directly beneath a stop marked with a blue bus.
- ➤ He needs a coffee. Bus drivers do this. I asked once for coffee… didn't go over well… I digress…

So my driver, my guide, my employee of the public transportation system has no worldly clue where I am going. My schedule said I should get there by 8:30. I figure about 10 minutes prior I will start looking for it.
The time quickly turns to 8:20am. I move myself to the front of the bus to try to look at cross streets.

I decide to ask the rag tag group of strangers on the bus if they know where the high school is. They don't. Just like a beam of light a man sits next to me and tells me he walks past the high school on his way to his brothers. I could get off with him and he will guide me. I have an hour before the race. I have to follow him.

We get off the bus and he says it's going to be a little while because the school is about a mile away. Whatever! I'm going to do a 5k, who cares about this one little mile? Not me. We walk and he's very kind. He shows me the school and keeps on walking. There are some kids playing soccer in the field and there is a man doing lawn maintenance.

"Can you direct me to the track?" I ask with the absolute confidence that I am in the right spot.

"The track?" He looks confused or he's looking at me like I'm confused.

"Yes. I'm here for the 5k, this is the high school, right?" As I speak I'm noticing that for a 5k there's very few people milling about.

"Oh no, this is the middle school. But you're close."

"Oh, good! How do I get there?" Close is good.

"Where are you parked?"

Parked? Now I definitely look confused. "I didn't drive."

"Oh! You are NOT close." He squelches a laugh.

Now, I'm holding my breath. "How far?"

"It's about 2 miles or so to Annaquatucket Road, then you take a left and go at least another half a mile or so to the road the school is on."

"Okay, thank you. Looks like I need to get going."

I'm completely lost but determined to make this 5k. I decide to start my jog so I can make it in time. People that consistently drive have no real concept of mileage so I was positive it was closer than that. I take off heading back the way I arrived. I saw the man that wrongly told me where I was going.

"What are you doing back here?" He asks.

"That was actually the middle school."

His face contorts. "Oh, yeah, it is. Sorry."

"No worries, I know where I'm going now."

I pass him. Felt nice to pass him even if he was walking. I wasn't walking. I liked that. So I make my way to Annaquatucket and turn left. I keep going.

And going.

And going.

I'm now beginning to doubt where I am. I have been jogging for quite some time. Just when I thought all was lost, I saw the sign that indicated the school was up ahead.

I was wearing a sweatshirt during all of this in 85 degree weather! I did that because I wanted to be able to feel cool when I started running by making myself hot at the get go. I ended up turning into the school with 5 minutes to spare already drenched in sweat.

I get to the entry table and get my number. 36. Darn! I really wanted 35 since it was my birthday but there was no time to complain, I needed to get out there.

In my training I have been hesitant to go more than 4 miles at a time. I think that once I get to that point my shins begin to hurt and so do my feet. By the time I started the race I was beyond all of that. I had no pain, no fear, I was ready!

I jogged for as long as I could and then decided I had to speed walk the rest of the course. I got to see a beautiful town that I hadn't been to in years. I got to smell wild grapes which always brings back memories of my grandfather when he would take me fishing by river near our house. It was wonderful.

I was happy with my first mile time considering how much running I had already done before the race even started. I checked my watch and I was looking for my mile 2 time. There were plenty of flaggers but none that were giving me the mile marks. I just kept plugging away and really beginning to doubt my internal time and ability to do a mile. It just seemed so long.

Before I knew it I was back at the school. They only showed the marker for the first mile and none of the others. I was so concerned about mile 2 that I didn't realize I completed mile 2 AND 3! There was an Olympic style finish so when we returned to the school the finish line was on the track. Once I hit the track I saw the time. It was 14 minutes faster than my previous time! The most surprising thing was that I could've gone longer.

When I got home I Googled where I got off the bus and realized that I jogged 5 MILES BEFORE THE 5K!

Here are some valuable lessons I learned on the morning of my 35th birthday:

> Just put one foot in front of the other and not obsess over mile 2 or any other things along the way

> My physical limitations are self-imposed. I have the power to physically do more than I ever imagined. If you asked me Friday how far I could jog I would have said 2 miles strong. That is no longer true.

> The high school used to be behind the middle school I originally went to, they built a new school just a couple of years ago so Wrong Direction Guy wasn't totally wrong.

> I should really start driving again.

My next major run was the Hyannis Half Marathon in February 2008. It was 5 months away. I was scared to death.

Those months passed like wild fire! What was I doing? I booked my entry into the Hyannis Half Marathon back in July after finishing the corporate challenge 5K in Boston where I was clearly still under the influence of Runners High!

As much as I wanted my children and my parents to see me cross the finish line, I also didn't want to fail in front of the people I love the most. Thirteen miles is a long way for healthy people and even though I trained for this I was still 330lbs and had no idea if I could pull this off. I set out for the race completely alone.

I got to Hyannis, Massachusetts, by bus on Saturday afternoon. The run start was early in the morning so I went to the Marathon Expo to pick up my race packet. There were tons of dealers selling everything in the world that have to do with running. Gloves, thermals, performance fleece, shoes, you name it. It was overwhelming.

I finally made my way through the expo to where I would get my race packet. It contains my number, my timing chip, and basic information. All the names of the runners were tacked on the wall and it looked like thousands of people were going to run on Sunday. Looking around everyone seemed to look like athletes. Like serious athletes. And then there was me. I don't look like a marathon runner... not even a half marathon runner but when I picked up my packet they looked at me like an athlete. That eased a lot of my tension.

Did you know that there's a division for heavier runners? I didn't know until I registered. The terms and weight limits vary but for this race the term is Filly for women and Clydesdale for men. Yes, horse names. How heavy do you have to be to be in the Filly division for this race? A whopping 140lbs. I was technically more than TWO Filly runners. My tension returned.

I saw that I was properly listed in the Filly division but I wasn't sure if I needed to weigh in somewhere. There were so many people that I wasn't even sure who to ask. The line was blurred since everyone had 2% body fat and running gear on from the racers, the vendors, and the staff. I turn to the woman next to me and decide to bite the bullet and ask her.

"Excuse me, ma'am, where do I go for weigh in for the Filly division."

"Oh, there's no weigh in. It's more of the honor system," she said.

Looking back on that conversation years later I realize just how kind she was to me. Since the Filly Division weight limit started at 140lbs and I was clearly well above that, she could've said some horrendous or snarky things but she was very gracious. Truth be told, runners are the most supportive people I've encountered in sports.

I tried to get over my Two Filly status and started to feel completely out of my league. Should I even be here? I could easily just go back to my hotel room and hide there until this is over. I am not a runner and from the looks of everyone around me I'm never going to be one either.

I went to the tables to put my stuff down and look in the packet. The crowd was starting to concentrate to the front. I was curious to see what was happening there. I saw two people that I wasn't expecting but nearly made me cry on sight. Rick & Dick Hoyt were there at the front of the room signing books.

Rick & Dick Hoyt are a father and son team of endurance athletes like you have never seen before. I can barely type this without wanting to cry and to be able to meet them in person was just inspiring. Dick Hoyt didn't start running until he was quite advanced in age and he pushes his on in a specialized chair the entire marathon. Team Hoyt has also done the Ironman Triathlon where father Dick swims 2.4 miles with his son in a boat, then rides on a bike with his son in a special seat for 112 miles and

THEN does a complete 26.2 mile marathon. I've seen them on TV a bunch of time and I couldn't believe they were here!

I was at the end of the line and that was the best thing ever. I was fortunate to be able to speak to them for over half an hour and Dick even signed my copy of his book. I felt like I had all the inspiration that I could need to get me through the day. If a man in his sixties could push his 45 year old son all the way then I can do this. I trained for this. I got this!

On Sunday morning I woke up to 28 degrees two days after a snow storm and was prepping for my 13.1 mile run. I was dressed in layers and the cutest hat that read: I RUN LIKE A GIRL. I felt fierce and ready. I get to the start and I feel invincible. Then I look around. Everyone is stretching and prepping and I'm just standing there. People are putting Vaseline on their feet. WHAT? My anxiety starts to rise again. I had to keep telling myself that I can do this. I trained to do this. I got this. The Hyannis Marathon is a qualifying race so there were plenty of runners who were vying for a coveted qualifying time for the Boston Marathon and they weren't there to play. I just wanted to finish my half marathon alive. That was my only goal: Cross the finish line alive.

The shot goes off and we take off. I feel good and it's cold but bearable. Every runner will tell you to dress in layers and not anything you love because these cold start races you'll start to peel off your layers and abandon them on the course. Within the first mile I saw gloves, then jackets, then pants. I was convinced everyone ahead of me – which was everyone – will be completely naked by the finish.

The first 3 miles were an absolute breeze. My first 5k back in July seemed like a miracle to complete and now I did three miles before it even registered. I felt strong and surprisingly confident.

The course is a loop so the full marathoners do the loop twice but the half marathoners do the loop one time. The 10k runners are doing just over six miles so at the six mile mark the 10k group splits off from the rest of the pack to their finish line. I was very proud of myself because I felt FABULOUS at that point. I blew a kiss to the 6 mile marker and mentally said so long to the 10k group. I couldn't believe I was actually out here doing this and doing it well.

That was until Mile 9 where I was apparently hit by a speeding train. At least that's what it felt like. I've heard the phrase "hit the wall" a million times in my life but I never felt it before Mile 9. I know what it feels like now. I felt like my energy supply was gone and that my right foot was on fire. My brain was telling me that no one would care if I quit and the only thing I really wanted was to be airlifted out of there immediately. I knew for a fact that if I got on the ground the ambulance would be there in moments to deliver me to the finish. It was tempting. So tempting.

Then I thought of my son who wrote me a note that I kept in my pocket that read "Be safe, run hard, I love you." I thought of my daughter who started this whole running thing when she picked up the Nicoderm last April and insisted I quit. I thought of the readers of my blog who have always been so supportive. I didn't want to let anyone down.

Then my mental game started to come back. I didn't train so hard to stop. I didn't run in 20 degree weather to go all the way out there and then go home. I wanted to finish this race. With my burning right foot, I got my resolve back and trudged on.

I literally trudged. People doing the half marathon and the marathon were starting to drop out of the race by this point.

Then the elite runners started coming around on their second lap. I was embarrassed but when you can run and entire marathon in less than three hours they were bound to pass me. I thought that they would yell for me to get out of the way. And they did yell.

"You're doing great! Keep going!"

"Hang in there honey, you can do it."

"You are my inspiration."

Just hearing them say these words, I was instantly returned to my life before running. This time last year I barely walked from the couch to the fridge. I smoked cigarettes like Philip Morris cut me a check to smoke for them. I ate myself into insanity and NEVER for one second of my life did I think that I could accomplish something so huge. Just when I needed my mental game to get back on the elite runners came and gave me all the encouragement I needed.

At Mile 10 a young woman ran along side of me.

"Hey, are you okay?" She asked.

"Yes, I'm fine," I lied. I was hardly fine. I felt like I was dying. She was wearing a marathon relay bib so she was doing a leg of the marathon as part of a team. I was jealous.

"Want me to run with you?" She asked me clutching her baton.

"No, I'm fine. I don't want to disrupt your team."

"It's okay," she was very cheerful as I assume someone would be during their first couple of miles.

"Thank you, really, but I'm ok. Go ahead and crush this with your team."

"You're doing great, keep up the good work!" She ran ahead and I was grateful for the chat.

It took me what seemed like forever to do those last 3 miles. But with my burning foot and my "I Run Like a Girl" hat I crossed the finish line. There at the finish was the Mile 10 buddy with her marathon relay team. She waited to see me at the finish and she was probably there for an hour! I was so happy but once I ran into the finish chute I lost her. To this day I have no idea who she is but if she ever reads this I need her to know that I will be eternally grateful for her and her team cheering me on at the finish.

It took me over 4 hours to finish. Far longer than I thought it would take but I didn't set out to make records, or win awards. I set out to cross the finish line alive and I did. Let the record reflect that I did finish BUT I was dead last. DEAD LAST. There were 1823 people doing the Half Marathon that day and I finished in 1823rd place. I was happy I finished but that did take a little wind out of my sails.

Once I got back to my hotel I did the craziest thing. I went to the fitness center and I got on a stationary bike. I read an article about the benefits of continuing to move after a long run. After 20 grueling minutes I went to my room and crashed until morning.

I opened my eyes in the pre-dawn hours and hoped that I could walk! I had to catch an early bus and was going directly to work. I was able to walk just fine but the blister on my foot was pretty bad. As I tried to gently put in my foot in my shoe my toenail fell off.

Another casualty of running war. I learned much later that the Vaseline that everyone was swabbing everywhere was to prevent blisters and toe nail loss. A great mystery solved albeit too late.

I got on the bus and headed back to Providence with my finisher's medal in hand. I was feeling better about the finish because I finished and that was what I wanted. Then came the perspective I needed. We passed a road sign in Seekonk, MA, that read:

T.F. Green Airport 12 Miles

Rhode Island is a small state but I was in Massachusetts and the airport is in the middle of the state in Warwick! My disappointment quickly melted and the true feeling of accomplishment was finally there. I ran (and walked, and cried) farther from where I was on the bus to the AIRPORT! That is accomplishment!

CHAPTER FIVE
INTRODUCING LOVE & MOPEDS

I was always quick with wit. I'm the type of person that can have a snappy come back and make you laugh instantly. I was particularly good at self-deprecating humor. It was far easier to make a funny comment about my weight before you could make one about me. It would diffuse the tension or discomfort that I always felt because I was usually the largest person in a room. Make a joke, everyone laughs, we move on. It worked for decades.

Every time I laughed at myself it was usually to cover just how uncomfortable I was, how embarrassed I was, and how ashamed I was. I could never stick to any diet or any program with any success. Even though I was happy in so many areas of my life my weight was always my albatross. When you spend a lifetime not liking something so obvious about yourself you start to believe the lies that you've told yourself for years:

I'm not worthy.

I'm not good enough.

No one is going to love me like this.

I remember talking to one of my friends who was dating a man who never took her out. They would always stay in and watch movies, eat delivery, and spend time alone. Usually at night. At the end of a long day. You get me. After several months of being with him and never going anywhere she decided to ask him about going out. He replied:

"Dating fat women is like riding a moped. Fun to ride but you don't want to be seen on one."

Imagine hearing that. Imagine someone saying that to you. How would that feel? As a big woman that's another fear. People will use you. Use you for your kindness, your money, your access, whatever you have that they can abuse.

That story made every single person in my life a suspect. If a man is interested in me what is he really interested in? Makes you think. It also made me stay home. I had enough horrible relationships in my day. I wasn't ready to venture back out into the storm of dating. Who wants to face that kind of disappointment? Then an event happened that made me remember that I was alive and forced me to go out again.

There was a large cancer charity hosting an event that fall and the company I worked for set up a corporate team. I wanted to be a part of it. I wanted to do something to honor my cousin Sybil but asking people for money was not my strength. How can I raise money but not ask for it? I used to sing so I decided to put on a "mini-concert" and have a basket raffle. If I can get enough people from work to go and get decent items donated, we can raise the money to reach our goal and I don't have to ask anyone.

One of the men who just started working with me was a karaoke DJ and he volunteered to do the music. Within a couple of days, we had the venue, the donated items, and the music. We were officially an event and had 4 months to get everything together. The DJ also told me that he and his wife host karaoke at this little bar outside the city every Wednesday night and if I wanted to practice I could head over there one night.

The following Wednesday, another coworker and I decided to go and give it a shot. She also likes to sing too so it would be a fun night. I walk in the door and the hosts are already there setting up. They know everyone in the place. Next to the DJ table there were high top tables and barstools and there was a man wearing a cowboy hat sitting at the closest table to them. When they introduced us to Jeff I'll never forget how I felt. He was tall sitting down and when I extended my hand out to shake his I looked into his eyes and I was immediately taken to the movie The Princess Bride. Buttercup described Wesley as having "eyes like the sea after a storm." That's exactly what I saw. We sat with him and talked all night. Jeff was more than tall cowboy with incredible eyes, he could sing. Whoa, could he sing. Amazing. Simply amazing.

To say that I liked him right away would be an understatement. He was kind and funny and we laughed a good portion of the night. There weren't many singers that night, so we had several opportunities to sing and that was a lot of fun.

This bar had a nice way to encourage people to sing. Each person would get a raffle ticket after every song they sang and at the end of the night you could win a $50 gift certificate to the bar. That could pay for your evening! The hosts pull the winning ticket and Jeff was the winner. The table next to us had a large group of women who were celebrating one of their friends moving away. They were having a great time the entire night. As soon as they called Jeff's name and he won he walked that $50 gift certificate to them and told them have fun. They were stunned. He just smiled and walked back to our table. I thought that was really sweet. This was the beginning of my friendship with cowboy Jeff.

The entire summer leading up to the event in October we hung out most Wednesdays singing. He was always kind and respectful and although he was nearly 8 years older than me I never felt like we weren't able to be good friends. He worked in computers and when my laptop was on the fritz he offered to come over and take a look at it. He was just finishing up dinner and said he'd be right over.

I was standing in my living room in an oversized t-shirt and leggings with a pair of my daughter's tall striped toe socks without my toes in the toe parts because it's horribly uncomfortable. I was so nervous he was coming to my house! Should I change my clothes? Should I do my hair? Should I put on makeup? I should be doing something! I freaked out for about 20 minutes and decided to do nothing. Who am I kidding? I've known Jeff for several months and if he was really interested in me he would have said something by now. Why would a tall, blue-eyed cowboy with a singing voice to die for be interested in me anyway? I settled back into my reality and waited for him to arrive.

He showed up as promised and I'm ever the picture of toe-socked loveliness. He was barely in the door when he got a phone call. The next 15 minutes was so awkward. He was on the phone having a conversation that seemed like computer information mixed with personal small talk. I wanted to crawl in a hole. After he hung up I foolishly asked a question, "Who was that?" He foolishly responded, "A girl I should probably be dating."

I don't think the look on my face could properly showcase how I felt inside. At least I no longer had to waste another moment on the Does He Like Me Game. That was a deep resounding no. Loud and clear. We talked as he fixed my virus laden computer. By the time he left I was happy. He's a nice guy and a good friend. Just as he was before. Knowing that he isn't interested in me shouldn't change that fact. Again, why would he like someone like me anyway?

We hung out more frequently and it was almost time for the event. We actually had two events planned back to back for the cancer fundraiser. The first event was Friday night and one of the guys at work had a band. This really cool bar would allow bands to play and charge $5 per person to get in and for the fundraiser we got all the door money and they just hope people buy drinks and food. In Rhode Island, most bars outside of the city close at 1am but the bars in the city close at 2am. Every Friday night Jeff and his friends would sing at a restaurant in Cranston that closed at midnight. As I was in the bar playing host for the fundraiser I decided to call Jeff to see if he wanted to meet me in the city for this fundraiser. To my surprise, he said yes.

Jeff lived about 15 minutes from the city and - somehow - had no idea how to get around. I tried to give him directions to where I was, and he was driving in circles for a very long time. I finally told him to stop and park and I will find him. He parked and started walking and I left the bar to meet him. As I'm walking down the street, a manhole cover has steam coming out from it clouding the alley. The streetlights cast an ominous glow and then I see him emerge from the steam like out of a Hollywood movie. Standing 6'5" he looks nearly 7 feet tall in cowboy boots and a hat and when he sees me I go to hug him and he kissed me! This was not the kiss of a friend, this was not the kiss of a man who had someone who should be his girlfriend! What was this? What did it mean? I didn't care, I just kissed him back.

We settled into the bar listening to the bands, kissing, and talking for the next couple of hours. I learned more details about his life, his family, his children and he learned about mine. He's the fifth of six children and I'm the sixth of seven so we had a lot of commonality with big families. We talked about our children and how we both started having children at age 22. It was always so easy to talk to him and that didn't change at all. It was really nice to be so comfortable with him.

After the fundraiser was over and the bar was closing he drove me home and I had to ask the million-dollar question, "How long have you wanted to kiss me?" My brain was already preparing itself for disappointment and that I seriously misread what was happening here. He replied, "Since I met you." I called absolute shenanigans! "You said that you should be dating the girl on the phone at my house!" He claimed he had no idea why he said that, and he was so concerned that since he was older than me that I wouldn't be interested in him. Here I was thinking that because of my size he wouldn't find me attractive. Oh, how the insecurities of our minds can ruin everything.

The following night was the fundraiser that we worked on for months. I would sing and so would some of my friends. We had great gift baskets, a beautiful venue, and a mission to raise money for our team. When Jeff and I showed up that night our friends knew something had changed with us. We let them know that we were seeing each other, and they were stunned but happy. He got to meet most of my coworkers and everyone seemed to see in him what I saw in him. Not just his kindness but that he really made me happy. We were always friends now it was something deeper.

I decided to surprise Jeff with tickets to see the Big Men of Country Concert but the closest location was in Buffalo, New York, about eight hours from where we were. I made the plans to have a couple of hotel rooms and take the kids with us for our first road trip adventure. We decided to leave at night, so we could drive all night and wake up in Buffalo! Great plan. I'm a bit nervous in the car and I frequently hit my imaginary brake. I can be a bit much to deal with in the car. I took some Nyquil and we took off. Jeff driving, me riding shotgun, with Darienne, Samantha, and Nicholas in the backseat of the Buick. This was going to be fun.

I remember at one point through my Nyquil addled brain hearing Nicholas talk to Jeff about the mountains. I chucked to myself because the Berkshires are more like "mountains" when compared to actual MOUNTAINS. Then I drifted back to sleep.

I woke up to Nicholas talking about seeing the Canadian flag in the distance and I let him know that Buffalo is close to Toronto, so it wouldn't be uncommon to see Canadian flags. We decided to take a break and get a bit to eat at a local McDonald's. Jeff was grateful to stop because he was driving for nearly 8 hours. We were all so excited to be in Buffalo and immediately after breakfast took off to find our hotel.

We were only on the road for a few minutes before we stumbled upon the Canadian border! There was a large sign that read "If you aren't going to Canada keep right." We were not going to Canada so we took the hard right into the duty-free shopping area at the border. Jeff and I headed inside to find out where we were and to get better directions to the hotel.

We tell the first worker we see that we're looking for Buffalo and we needed to know how far away we were. She looked extremely confused and said she had to get her manager. We were also confused that directions would require management but soon enough the manager came over.

"You guys looking for Buffalo?" He asked.

"Yes, we are. About how far away are we? Jeff asked.

"I bet you used Google Maps. Come one, we got to go to the big map."

At this point we are thoroughly confused. We needed to walk to a big map?

Why? We follow him around a corner and there's a huge map hung on the wall.

He pointed to Buffalo and said, "You're looking to go here. But you are right here."

He points to the top of the map by MONTREAL! What? That was the day we learned that Google Maps 2008 had a bit of a snafu around Albany and we were one of many humans how took the wrong turn and drove 7 hours in the wrong direction. In my head I'm replaying the conversation Nicholas had with Jeff about "mountains" and he really saw   MOUNTAINS...   Adirondack Mountains!

We had no idea what we were going to do. The plan was to spend the day in Niagara and then go to the concert. We had to figure out how to get to the concert! Our new friend gave us two options. The first one involved back tracking to Albany and I was not a fan of that. The next one was that we could take these little country roads and hug the Canadian border all the way to Buffalo. He was getting off work in 15 minutes and if we were willing to wait he could guide us to the road we would need to take. We blindly followed a perfect stranger down the road for several miles before he waved us to the road.

For the next 8 hour we see things we never would've seen if our original plan worked out. We saw countless tiny villages and stretches of beautiful farmland, an enormous wind turbine farm that stretched acres, and every single tiny hamlet in upper New York. It was beautiful, and we had fun.

We made it to the concert only missing the first opening act and the following day experienced true upstate New York weather. When we entered Niagara it was a seemingly beautiful fall day. Within an hour it was snowing, followed by sunshine, and then rain. Our pictures from that afternoon look like we spent a week in Niagara with one set of clothes. We were exhausted but we made our way back home without incident.

When we returned I knew that I was going to be with Jeff forever. There's no way anyone else on earth could get so lost for so long and me not want to kill them! The following Monday at work he had flowers delivered to me with this card: It was a pleasure getting lost with you. From that day forth, we were inseparable. We would talk all the time and he was an expert at making me laugh with his never-ending stream of lame jokes. The kids even took pretty well to him. If you would have asked me 5 years prior if I would be dating a tall, cowboy I would've laughed. I don't like country music, not my style, and I would have staked something pretty sacred that it wouldn't happen. I would've missed one of the great joys of my life.

One of the most challenging parts of our relationship was my perception of it. I would still have these horrible thoughts in the back of my mind about if he really liked me. He said all the right things, did all the right things, and there I was in my head trying to figure out why someone like him would want to be with someone like me. I kept thinking of the moped discussion. I never shared these thoughts with Jeff, I would just silently think them and try to drown them in ice cream.

We were not without challenges in the first few months of our relationship but one of the biggest indictors that this was going to be different was how we related to each other. In my past relationships, I would have a tendency to use my sharp wit mixed with a sharper tongue when I'd fight. I noticed with Jeff that no matter how frustrating the situation I never would throw a disarming jab. I cared about him too much to do that.

Another interesting thing was that no matter how hard I tried to push him away and challenge if he really loved me he never shied away from me. It was the most comfort I had ever felt and it was something so hard to get used to.

Within months we moved in together. As time drifted on, Jeff was like a lighthouse beacon in a storm. As the sea raged around me emotionally when I looked to him I found a sense of peace, safety, and hope. It would be some time before we both realized the true Lighthouse.

CHAPTER SIX
SHEDDING FOR THE WEDDING... AND OTHER LIES

It was a beautiful night and we were at this restaurant in Exeter, Rhode Island, on karaoke night. Any other night would've been foolish. We met singing and it made perfect sense that he would propose to me while singing. I had no idea that it was going to happen.

When the DJ called his name and he went up to sing it was just like any one of the hundreds of times he's walked to a mic to sing. As he finished Clay Walker's love song Fall he asked me to come to the front and he presented me with a ring and in front of the entire restaurant asked me to be his bride.

I was overjoyed and so happy. I've loved Jeff since we met and it didn't change after a year of living together. We only got stronger together. I was ecstatic to be his wife. I never dreamed I would be married and to be married to Jeff would be a dream come true.

When initial excitement started to wane and I could begin the actual planning of the wedding I was stuck with a paralyzing thought. I was over 350lbs and I did NOT want to be a heavy bride. I had to start dieting immediately. We decided to get married in October 2011, so I had two good years to get my eating and weight under control. I had plenty of time. Famous last words.

The first round of dieting took place with just focusing on eating properly. I joined Weight Watchers and was doing pretty well. My meeting was in Johnston, RI, and it consisted of many wonderful older ladies who liked to socialize and lament over the 8lbs they wanted to lose before St. Joseph's Day so they could eat 10 zeppoles without guilt. Needing to lose so much weight made me feel really out of sorts with this group. They were all very kind and the leaders were great but I just didn't find any traction there. I took my membership online and I liked it. There was a lot of support from likeminded people and I was able to engage with blogs and forums. I did well for a while.

My problem has always been being honest

with myself about my weight. I don't know who I thought I was lying to or how it would help me but there I was trying to game another weight loss system and wondering why it wasn't working.

First, I would just not enter some of the food I ate. Obviously, if you don't write it down it didn't happen and those calories didn't exist at all. Then at weeks end I was shocked and horrified that I didn't lose any weight – or worse – gained it. Next, I would falsify my stats so I wouldn't be judged by any of my online WW friends.

I maintained this appearance until it was too painful to continue making weekly payments and weekly fabrications and not have anything to show for it. Back to the drawing board. I went back to trying to be more responsible with what I ate and how much I ate.

Jeff was always very supportive of my efforts but having joint accounts made it so that he could see where I was eating so he'd question me about my choices. When McDonalds would appear in my online banking he'd ask about my dieting. It got to the point where having cash was like the biggest thrill in the world! I could eat ANYWHERE with cash and however much I wanted. No questions, no judgments, no problem.

Focusing on losing weight only made me more anxious about my weight which in turn made me uncomfortable about my weight, which was only made better by eating. Vicious circle, indeed. Then I'd follow that up with lying about what I was eating and where and the mental toll was excruciating but it continued on.

Having opportunities for cash was few and far between so I developed a new plan with my debit card. I would find "safe places" where I could buy the things I wanted without judgement or detection. I frequently go to dollar stores or convenience stores and it was easy to slip a couple of candy bars in with my normal purchases. No questions! I just had to destroy the receipts before I got home.

These antics reminded me of when I was living alone and ordering take out. I would always order an obnoxious amount of food but I was sure to pretend like I was ordering for multiple people so they wouldn't think that one person was going to eat all of that food. I'm sure they knew it was just me and they probably didn't care but it was important to me to have that illusion. My favorite was ordering two large Italian subs and making sure one had extra mayonnaise and oil and vinegar. I would then have them put Rob on the sub with the extras so we could tell them apart. Rob is my brother and I've never consumed a single Italian sub with him in my life but according to our local take out place we ate together frequently. Ridiculous .

I'm trying to get a handle on my food consumption and I did lose some weight but with every loss there another gain right around the corner. It was abundantly obvious that my weight was just spiraling out of control when we took the kids to Hull, MA, for February vacation in 2010.

The beach in Winter is one of my favorite sights. Going up to Hull with the kids was just a way for us to get away when school was out and spend some time together. We booked connecting rooms so we all had some privacy but the only caveat with connecting rooms is that they only connected double bed rooms at this hotel. We were fine with that until we got into a double bed.

When Jeff and I met he was sleeping diagonally on a queen bed since he's 6'5" tall and his ankles would hang off the bed. The double beds were full size beds which are fine for most people not people like Jeff and me.

We crawl into bed that first night and discover with my well over 300lb frame and his tall stature we were best served sleeping separately. I didn't want to go on vacation and sleep separately.

I could barely sleep that first night. Sleep is usually hard for me to come by anyway but our sleeping arrangements really upset me. Why can't I get a handle on this? What is my problem? I went to the vending machine and got various snack cakes to help me think of why I can't get my life together.

The following months were more of the same. Try this. Try that. Do this. Do that. Eat this. Eat that. All to no avail because I couldn't stay out of my own way long enough to really face what was happening. I managed to lost about 50lbs but I was really hoping for more before the wedding. By March of 2011, I needed to commit to a dress and I was running out of time.

My biggest fear with dress shopping was going somewhere and they wouldn't have anything that fit me. I've seen those shows where they wedge a woman into a sample dress that's way too small but fill the gaps in with tablecloths and industrial clips. I was not trying to having that experience.

One of Jeff's friends was dating a woman

who worked as a sales associate at David's Bridal and I liked her. She was always really nice and upbeat. My level of freak out was growing longer but my time was running shorter so I sent her a message asking if she could show me some gowns and I shared my concern about my size. She was so gracious and was happy to take my appointment. She even assured me that there were dresses of all sizes that I could try.

I decided to keep my appointment with her privately even though every single dress show has a full entourage of woman all crowding around the blushing bride offering all kinds of commentary. That sounded horrifying to me. There was no way I was involving anyone in this process. I could be embarrassed alone but to share that with friends or family was out of the questions.

The night before my appointment my emotions were at an all-time high. I had no idea how this was going to go and I was actually nervous to do it alone. I called my friend Pam who lived in Rhode Island but as far away as you can get in our tiny state and still call it RI. I was in a panic about my appointment and I asked if she could come. I let her know that I was planning to just go it alone but I really needed her there. She agreed and we met the following afternoon.

Dress shopping is overwhelming. You go in with a thought of what you want and what you think will look good on you. Sometimes those two things are mutually exclusive. I remember seeing a dress in a magazine that I liked but it had everything I hated: lace, beads, sleeveless, and strapless. I had no idea why I liked that dress but on the size 2 model it did look extraordinary. I decided to start with what I wanted to hide. Clearly, my arms needed to be covered since I've never shown my arms in literally 30 years. Then I needed something to try to hide my stomach... as much as you can hide my stomach. As we roamed the aisles looking for things our attendant also had some ideas.

My first trip to the dressing room was an adventure. The undergarment to wear under formal wear is aggressive but what you wear under a wedding gown is simply brutal. The first gown was bright white, had long sleeves and a wide skirt. When I finally got in it and looked in the mirror I felt like a wall. One enormous wall. On the center of the sun. I decided the bright white was not an option and The saleswoman suggested something with a shorter sleeve to give some break in the dress. She also said it will be slenderizing as well. I can be sold with slenderizing!

Every single dress had a problem. Too much skirt, too much skin, too much, not enough, etc. I was never going to find something that I like that worked with me. Honestly, it was none of the dresses. Ultimately, I wasn't happy with the body going in the dresses not the dresses themselves. I was trying not to cry in front of my friends. This was so disappointing,

On my final trip into the aisles I found a dress that was similar to the dress I liked from the magazine. It was champagne with ruching, beads, and was sleeveless. Surely to look horrendous on me but so did everything else. We were getting close to the end of my appointment so this was going to be my last shot.

When I put the dress on something happened. I felt pretty good but my arms were exposed and my there was a lot of detail and attention to my waist. How was I not freaking out? This was the first dress I wanted to see myself in the tree panel mirror. As I go out I see Pam's face change. She liked it . I stood in front of the mirror and I was so surprised at how good I felt. After she placed the veil on my head, I felt like a bride for the first time. Those wedding TV shows may have some corny moments but when you add a veil things really do happen.

As beautiful as it was and as beautiful as I felt I still couldn't commit that moment. I needed my mother to see it. I made another appointment with my friend for later in the week and invited my mom to see the dress.

The new appointment day was upon us and I was already stressed out. What if it doesn't feel the same today? What if something new came out and I would want that? What if my mother doesn't like it?

I got there early and decided to take another trip through the aisles to see if there was anything I may have missed. I pulled a couple of items to try with my other gown.

My first trip in the dressing room was with a sleeveless ball gown with a full skirt and sweetheart neckline. I was hoping the fullness of the skirt would make my waist smaller. It did not. Not at all. I was back to feeling like a wall. Maybe this wasn't a good idea. I tried on quite a few more and nothing seemed to work.

My mother arrived and I just decided to put on my original dress because everything else seemed like a waste of time. Putting it on again was still magical. I felt so at home in it. I walk out of the dressing room to show my mother and I can see by her expression that she likes it too and I know that she was surprised to see my arms exposed. Just as I went to say something the woman who works in alterations walks by and looks me up and down.

"That is your dress," she said. She then continued on her way.

I was stunned. She has no vested interest in this process. She gets no commission from the sale of the dress and she doesn't know me from a hole in the wall. I loved that she said that. She sees women in dresses all day long and without warning or coaching she approved of my dress. I was ready to say yes.

Over the past few months, I was doing well with my weight loss and I had big plans to lose about 50 more pounds in the next 6 months but I had to order my dress that day because these things take time and I'd delayed as long as I could. I decided to do something to help me focus on those weight loss goals: I ordered my dress in a size 22 instead of the 26 I was wearing. If paying for the Half Marathon was a sure shot that I'd run, then paying way more money for a dress is all but a guarantee!

When my dress came in I declined trying it on when I picked it up. It had a corset back and I knew that I still had a bit of weight to lose but I was still confident I could make it work. I took the dress home and I tried to show Jeff the dress but he refused.

"It's so pretty! Don't you want to see it?" I taunted him.

He was adamant. "No, I'll see it when you walk down the aisle."

"But we aren't kids," I'd joke. "Come on, you know you want to see it."

"No, Regina, absolutely not."

Jeff was married before when he was very young and had 4 kids. His kids were all young adults by the time we got married and we even had grandkids. He had a simple wedding then and by this time was divorced for over a decade. I was never married but as I was approaching 39 years old with two kids these wedding traditions seemed a bit outdated to me. I kept the dress in its gusseted garment bag in an upstairs closet and I really wanted him to see it.

In all of the excitement of wedding planning there was one little thing I didn't count on that would make this process more difficult: stress. When I get stressed food was my great stress reliever, problem solver, anxiety treatment and elixir for any other emotion I didn't' want to feel. Planning a wedding is beyond stressful even for our small intimate gathering of just over 100 family members and friends. Between the invitations, venue, coordinating our six children, and everything else food became my everything. I knew I gained weight but I kept thinking I had time. Until time ran out.

The stress of knowing that there was no way I was fitting a dress 3 sizes smaller than the smaller size I was before was unreal. I would go up to the closet and look at the dress and wonder if there was anything I could do to make it work. I'm pretty handy with a sewing machine but working with a wedding gown is an entirely different skill. There's also the math of the situation. If something is too big you can arrange to have it taken in. If something is too small there has to be enough material to let out. This is all well and good for everyday clothes but the intricate design of wedding wear makes this a million times more challenging. My saving grace is that I picked a dress with a corset back so I was hopeful there would be enough room to work with and that the laces would be long enough to tie.

Two months before the wedding I called Pam and asked her to help me. I let her know that my weight and my gown size aren't quite matching up and I knew she would understand. She is also familiar with the roller coaster of weight. I stopped by a fabric store and picked up 3 yards of champagne colored satin. I wasn't sure what I would need or how I would do it but it definitely helped to start there.

She arrived and we ventured upstairs to the closet and I took out the dress. I had on my bridal corset and we put the dress on. The bad news was that the hook and eye that connected the corset sides at the top of the dress would NEVER connect even if I sucked in my gut until my spine showed. The good news was that the laces were long enough to go lace the entire back of the dress and tie.

When I took the dress off and looked at the back I saw that the piece that connected with the hook and eye was simply tacked to the back of the dress. I used a seam ripper and removed it with ease. I put the dress on again and this time we tucked the satin fabric into the top of my bridal corset and then laced the dress. It looked natural! I have never been so relieved. I tried to think of how many nights of sleep I lost wondering if I was going to have a dress to wear to my own wedding.

I celebrated with chocolate. Of course.

CHAPTER SEVEN
INTRODUCING ANOTHER LOVE

When I was a kid my first experience with Jesus was Vacation Bible School at the local Baptist church. It was not far from our house and we could actually trek through the woods and get there. We didn't' attend church there but my parents were thrilled that they would take all of us kids for several hours a day for an entire week in the summer. As a parent now I completely understand that logic.

I liked going to VBS. I was fascinated by the store of Shadrach, Meshach, and Abednego in the fiery furnace. I wanted to know more but my parents weren't too big on church. My father spent his entire childhood in church and what he remembers most is that he wanted to play baseball on Sunday's and their church was an all-day affair. Frequently, he'd sneak out the window of the church bathroom and go play baseball anyway. Every time he came home he could count on a solid whooping from my Grandfather. These memories don't spark an desire to take us to church.

My neighbor went to the local Catholic church and I started to attend with her. It was different from the Baptist church but I liked it. There was a sense of peace and pageantry that I really liked. I started to go as often as I could.

I went for several years until a turn of events when I was 12 years old changed my viewpoint on God. One of my friends was killed in a motor vehicle accident right in front of the church. I couldn't understand why God would allow such a thing to happen to someone who served him so faithfully. His parents were also active in the church and further complicating my relationship with God was that they only seemed to cleave closer to God after the loss of their child and I grew further away and was angry. By the time I was in high school God was way in my rear view mirror and I had no interest in seeking Him again.

My daughter started going to church with my mom's best friend. She liked to go and I was fine with her going. I didn't have to go. When Jeff and I started dating one of the first conversations we had was about faith and we were both perfectly fine in our lives without God in it.

When our friend's daughter was going to be in the church play we decided to go to support her. Darienne was going too so it was nice to have her see us support the church in our own way.

I've always loved plays and this play was amazing. It was geared for adults and it took place immediately following the rapture. As a "recovering Catholic" the only information I had about the rapture was from the Left Behind series of books that I didn't read but heard a lot about. The play really moved me and I wasn't prepared for it. I wanted to know more.

At the conclusion of the play one of the pastors came to the front of the stage and asked if anyone wanted a *New Believer's Bible* and welcomed anyone to see him after if they wanted more information. I wanted the *New Believer's Bible* but there was absolutely NO way I was walking up there in front of all of those people. I'll just go home and Google it.

The following week Darienne asked us to go to church. Since we both liked the play and this is the first time she's ever directly asked we decided to go. We climb in our friend's van and their granddaughter had a book for me. It was the New Believer's Bible! She said she wanted me to have it. I was stunned. How did this little girl know I wanted this Bible? She even filled out my name in the front and signed her name at the bottom! I was touched.

We get to the church and I have no idea what to expect. It's a large church by our local standards and that Sunday morning in April it was packed. We sat with our friends and the energy in the room was palpable. After a few brief announcements the band was on the stage and a large screen lowered and showed the lyrics to the songs they were singing.

I look over at Jeff, "Jesus Karaoke?" I whisper to him chuckling.

He smiles since he was thinking the same thing. This was definitely not a Catholic service in the 1980s. We used to have three hymns by number on a board and we'd all sing in quiet tones. Here people were standing, singing aloud, and really enjoying the music. The husband and wife team leading the singers had a joy that just filled the room. I had no idea what was happening but I knew I wanted more of it.

When we returned home I knew I needed to talk to Jeff. I liked what I experienced and I was wondering how he'd feel if I wanted to go again. I was a bit hesitant to have the conversation because we were both so strong in our desire to not have church in our lives and here I am getting ready to switch gears.

"What did you think of today?" I asked.

"I was surprised. I'm not sure what was happening but I liked it," he answered.

I was flabbergasted! "Would you want to go again?"

"I wanted to ask you," he said. "I just wasn't sure how you'd feel."

"That's exactly what I was thinking!"

We both agreed that we'd give it another try. Jeff was raised Episcopalian and had his own issues with church. We went back the following week and every week after that. That's how a former Catholic and former

Episcopalian who were living in sin started going to church.

As the months went by and we were already in the full on throws of wedding planning we were deepening our relationship with Christ. I poured through my New Believer's Bible eager to learn more. Our church offers a class called Face to Face that goes over their beliefs and how to grow in your faith. We offered to host the class at our home since it freed us of the burden of trying to get to the church since neither of us drove at that time. This was an incredible class. We learned so many things about Christ that we never knew as children and our hearts were incredibly opened.

Over the next few months we made an immense transformation in the way we lived and how we viewed all people. There was a genuine love and forgiveness for others but also for ourselves. We've both made mistakes in our lives that would eerily haunt us but we were able to give so much of that pain to Jesus and our lives were improved because of it.

Although we had been engaged for well over a year and lived together even longer I was starting to feel like it was improper that we lived together before we were married. We had less than a year before the wedding but with our going to church and taking immense strides with our faith I was feeling unsettled. Making the decision to adjust our lives to feel right with Christ as we prepared for marriage felt like what we needed to do. We decided to reside in the same home – since it was financially impossible to separate for just a few months – but to live as honestly and wholesomely as possible. Living a celibate lifestyle isn't impossible, but when you've lived a certain way for years and then you reverse the trajectory it can be a challenge. We were definitely challenged but we continued to learn, study, pray, and relate on a deeper level. It was a truly beautiful time.

We originally planned to be married by the ocean with a Justice of the Peace. Now, it seemed like a crazy thought to not be married by our Pastor. When he agreed to marry us we were elated! We started our Premarital Christian Counseling and we both still regard it as one of the greatest times in our togetherness. We learned a lot about each other but also about God's place in our lives and in our marriage. We agreed that if we always kept Jesus first then we were always on the same path. After this we had one piece of unfinished business.

The first time I accepted Christ through baptism I was 12 years old at my Catholic church. I was really behind schedule since everyone else was baptized as infants. Looking back I think it was important to me because everyone else was already baptized and I was the only one who hadn't received that sacrament. This time on that hot August afternoon I was in waist deep water and the reason I was there was not due to peer pressure or appearances or my desire to blend in. This time I was publicly proclaiming my faith and it was incredible. I heard somewhere that baptism is an outward pronouncement of an inward change. If you don't really feel what you believe then you're just getting wet. I have never felt so strong a belief in my life. Jeff was baptized immediately following me and we hugged in the pool. I felt such a feeling of love, hope, and faith in that hug. We were truly ready for marriage.

The final weeks of the wedding planning was absolute chaos. Plans made. Plans broken. RSVPs made. RSVPs cancelled. Financials all set. Financials all messed up. It was the most nerve-wracking time. It seemed like everything was absolute pandemonium. Adding to the insanity was that it was raining the night before the wedding. Not like regular rain but like a deluge.   Getting married in October in New England is a gamble. It could be beautiful with extended summer heat or it could be freezing. We've even had snow.

I awoke to a beautiful day. I didn't even look like it rained. Jeff was already up and gone before I could even see him. We had a lot of things to do still even though we got most of the decorating done before the rehearsal dinner the night before. It was the big day! Even though it was gorgeous outside it was still really windy so we decided to move the wedding inside but take pictures by the water after the ceremony.

Getting dressed was an adventure. I had a master plan. I decided to put on my bridal corset and then a layer of cling wrap followed by duct tape! I was going to tape away a good 50 pounds! Seemed like a genius plan. I was able to tape my way to a more tapered waist but that solution actually created two more problems: (a) I couldn't breathe... at all and (b) I couldn't sit.

What was I doing? Did I really think that I could tape away weight? Who was I trying to fool? Not a single person attending this event does not know that I am a heavy person and no amount of duct tape is going to hide that. As my mother, my daughter, and Pam remove the layers of tape I can hear the Holy Spirit clearly saying that Jeff loves me just as I am. I proceeded to finish getting ready and prepare to meet my father to walk me down the aisle.

My father took my hand and there was a small corner before we entered the ceremony. The look he gave me was priceless. My father and I had always been close and he's been my strongest support, the smartest man I've ever met, and one of the kindest souls ever. I know what a profound blessing it is to have a father especially one who was always so wonderful. Getting married at 39 to my very best friend was only made better by the fact that both of my parents were there to see it and that my father was able to walk me down the aisle.

As we turned the corner I looked at Jeff standing at the front of the room with our children and our best friends and when he saw me he immediately got tears in his eyes. I remember thinking of how many times I asked him to look at my dress and to think that if he did look I would've missed the look he gave me. I'm confident that no matter what my future holds I will never, ever forget the genuine look of love and awe that I saw on his face that day. I will forever be grateful that he wanted that traditional touch to our wedding.

The wedding was beautiful. Surrounded by our best friends and our children in our wedding party with our families in attendance was the greatest joy. Our friends who introduced us were so instrumental that day. Assisting with planning, last minute finances, and even pictures we owe them so much.

Everything felt sacred, holy, and blessed. Introducing Jesus into our lives elevated everything. I wanted to be a better wife, a better mother, a better person. I wanted to feel His divine presence every single day. We were already committed before our wedding but after that day we both changed for the better.

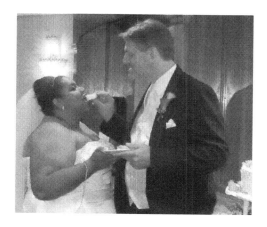

CHAPTER EIGHT
ANOTHER DAY ANOTHER DIET

Before the wedding I had lost 80 lbs and I walked down the aisle with 50 of them already back. By early 2012, I gained everything back with some additional for good measure. I was working at a startup company in Westerly, and almost every day I would eat at this Asian restaurant in town. The owner was really nice and would often let me order dinner size portions at lunch time. After months of visits she asked me for my phone number because she does lobster specials but not on set days. She was willing to call me and let me know when it was available. I thought that was so nice, I was happy to give her my number but I was quickly realizing that going out to lunch everyday was getting costly and foolish. I needed to get back on track.

I read an article online about how to break your habits and one suggestion was to establish your benchmarks. The secret was to analyze your habits now and then you can focus on setting a new pattern. Sounds good to me. For people looking for weight loss it was suggested that you take a week and just write down everything you eat. Every little thing! Then at the end of the week calculate how many calories you consumed. The goal was to see what you can remove right off the bat, then what you can pare down, and then what choices you can make better. They made it seem so simple. Write it down. Remove items that are no good for you, pare down larger portions of better things, and then substitute items like water for soda. Simple!

I wrote down everything I ate for a week. Just in the writing I started to notice that I eat a lot. Please let the record reflect that I knew I ate a lot but seeing it written down was a bit unsettling. I almost didn't write some things down but then caught myself trying to game the system again.

When it came down to figuring out the calories I attacked my list starting with Day One. I never did Day Two. After calculating

39,000 calories for my first day I was absolutely not going to further damage my psyche by looking at the rest. Horrified. Embarrassed. I couldn't believe it. Nutrition labels are calculated using a 2,000 calorie per DAY diet and I couldn't get past breakfast without breaking that. Olympic powerlifters can consume about 12,000 calories per day. I would do that by lunch time and my main activity was sitting. I didn't pick up that notebook again for months.

I continued my regular food behaviors and I continued to gain weight. I continued to be upset about it. I continued not doing anything to help myself. When I prayed about my weight I just prayed for God to fix it. I wanted to go to bed and wake up 150lbs. Why was that so hard? As sick as I was over the fact that my body that felt more like a prison than a temple, I continued to do nothing.

Facebook seems to store everything for eternity. One of my friends from college put up a Spring Break picture of me and one of my co-workers saw it. He asked me who that was and he couldn't believe it was me. He kept looking at this picture of me when I was at my lowest adult weight and looking at me now. All I could see in his expression was WHAT HAPPENED? He never said a word, his eyes said everything. I was so defeated.

A few days later I saw an advertisement for a ketogenic diet place that was opening near where I worked. It wasn't my first keto rodeo since I did have a bit of success at another medically supervised ketogenic diet when I worked in the city. I was intrigued. The ad featured huge letters across the top of the smiling After Picture of the model:

LOSE UP TO 100 POUNDS IN SIX MONTHS

Wow! That's a lot of weight in not a lot of time. I was definitely intrigued and now that our lives were settling in nicely maybe it was time to try again.

I spoke to Jeff when I got home and he was all for it. If I was happy he was happy. He's always been so supportive of everything I've ever done. I made the call and went for my consultation.

The consultation was actually presentation style and I was a little taken aback. I didn't want to discuss my weight in front of a bunch of strangers – or worse – people I knew. I sat in my car for a while then decided to bite the bullet and go in. The program was very similar to my last ketogenic program except it cost less weekly and had more food options. I was still getting B12 shots in my leg twice a week and weighing in once per week.

I liked the program and I also liked the office manager. She was really knowledgeable, friendly and kind. She made it easy for me to go every week and was just encouraging enough to make me continue. I did really well for quite a while. Jeff and I even started having fun preparing my lunches and making healthy dinners.

One day I received a voice message that I knew no one would believe and the outcome of that message was every harder to believe. The owner of the Asian restaurant called me and said this:

Hello Regina! How are you? I just wanted to call because you used to come in every day. Now you no longer come in. Did something happen? Do you not like my food anymore? What can I do to get you back?

I didn't call her back because I didn't know what to say and we always had a hard time understanding each other on the phone. About a week later I found myself heading to the same plaza that housed her restaurant. I planned to go in and say hello and show her my weight loss and explain where I've been.

I pulled into the plaza and the restaurant was now a tax filing place! She called a week prior and now the restaurant is closed and doing rapid refunds?

When I went home I told Jeff what happened and he didn't believe me. I let him listen to her message and then told him about how the restaurant was completely closed. Did I really eat so much that without me she had to close? I felt so bad I didn't call her back sooner.

Working for a startup had its disadvantages. When funding was low we weren't paid and it went from weeks to months. It was stressful but we were very optimistic because we really believed in the product but we also had bills to pay. Making things more difficult, was the fact that I was paying for my keto program weekly but I was continually missing paychecks. I continued with the program but we had to cut things in other areas to make it work.

When I reached the 6 months mark I had lost 75lbs. Seventy-five pounds. I distinctly recall being very upset. I remembered the ad:

LOSE UP TO 100 POUNDS IN SIX MONTHS

Here I was six months later out hundreds of dollars but not down hundreds of pounds.

With all the stress of not being paid and continuing to work and then NOT losing 100lbs I remember just being done. I was done with dieting. I was done missing bread. I was done eating broth and pretending I was happier without chocolate. I was not happy without chocolate. In fact, chocolate may very well be the definition of happy! Why was I doing this? It's cheaper to eat drive though dollar menu food and at least retain my sense of joy! I was done. Again. It didn't take long for my old food behaviors and volumes to return.

Heading toward the end of the year I was seeing a new primary care doctor. When I went into the exam room the nurse tried to weigh me on a scale that only went to 300lbs. I knew I was heavier than that. Here we go again.

When the doctor arrived he asked me if I ever considered weight loss surgery. I calmly said no. Inside I was SCREAMING! Did I look like I was that far gone? I can't believe he asked me that so casually. That's it. What could possibly be next?

CHAPTER NINE
VISUALLY DISTURBING

We were never people to go out for New Year's Eve even when we were drinking. Jeff had been sober for nearly a year on December 31, 2012, so going out was definitely not going to happen. My weight was still out of control and I'd been having some weird abdominal pains over the past few weeks.

Going to the doctor when you're overweight can be extremely frustrating. Many doctors can't see beyond your weight and think that if you were at a healthier weight then your ailments wouldn't exist. There may be some truth to that but there are times when an issue exists that has nothing to do with weight and will need to be addressed. I cringe thinking of going to the doctor.

On that clear New Year's Eve we were up

watching the ball drop. Most of our kids were home and we were having some sparkling apple cider to celebrate the occasion. Shortly after midnight I felt a sharp pain in my abdomen. That's not exactly accurate, it was more like I felt like I had been stabbed.

Jeff called 911 and I was dreading the next few things. Emergency workers will have to come in my house. They will attempt to lift me onto the gurney without dropping me. They will most likely try not to make me feel badly but will inevitably make me feel badly anyway. Then I will go to the hospital where the doctor will tell me that I'm fat and whatever my problem is would surely be cured with losing 150lbs. Ugh.

Jeff sat with me and held and my hands and prayed fervently for me. When the paramedic arrived it was almost like I was psychic. They fumbled getting me on the gurney and made large exertion noises getting me down the stairs. We got to the hospital in no time.

Since the doctors had no idea what was causing such acute pain they ordered an ultrasound an thought I may have a ruptured cyst on my ovary. My ovaries were fine. They then ordered an MRI.

Turned out my acute pain was cause by my

degrading uterus. It was in pretty bad shape but not bad enough to remove. I knew in 1996, that I was not ever going to have more children so I was a pretty strong advocate for a hysterectomy but I was declined. I had to have a procedure done but that's not the point of this story. After my hospital stay they gave me a DVD with my MRI to give to my doctor. I was curious so when I got home I popped it in my computer and I was absolutely horrified.

My organs looked "normal sized" then there was layer upon layer of fat. It was so clearly visible in the MRI. There was also fat around most of my organs. It was really awful to see. My doctor received a copy of the DVD from the hospital too so I was able to keep my copy. I tried to throw it away several times but I just couldn't bring myself to do it.

Some days when I was really down on myself I'd pop in the DVD and watch it... while eating ice cream.

What is it going to take to get my life together? I kept asking God to fix me but He never did. How could the God of everything not see that I really needed His help?

CHAPTER TEN
MY GUILTY VALENTINE

The startup company where I was working closed and I was at home drowning myself in ice cream at my disappointment that we didn't get funding in time to keep the company in Rhode Island.

After nearly falling down the stairs on New Year's Day 2014, I decided I had to do something. I wasn't sure what I was going to do but something had to give. I had so many wonderful things happening in my life and yet my weight was still keeping me from fully being happy and present. I was getting tired of being tired.

I kept seeing that image in my head of the picture my daughter took of me on the futon. I didn't want to look like that anymore. Perhaps it was time to look into weight loss surgery again.

My first venture into weight loss surgery was in 2002, when several of my friends was getting surgery. It was relatively new but once some high profile celebrities started having it and parading their new bodies all over television and magazines people were starting to pay attention. I was definitely paying attention.

I used to work with a woman who was a brilliant seamstress. She would whip up all kinds of things in no time. We were both quite overweight and I was grateful to have her in my department. We understood each other without having to say a word.

She was kind enough to use her awesome sewing skills to take a dress I wore from a summer wedding and put long sleeves on it so I could wear it on New Year's Eve. When it was ready I went to her house for a fitting and fine-tuning.

It was just before Christmas when I went to her house. She and her mother had fresh baked cookies everywhere. It smelled like heaven on earth! They were preparing for a holiday cookie swap and had already baked 30 dozen cookies!!!

One thing I noticed during that afternoon was that every time my friend went by the cooling racks she would eat a cookie. I wasn't even sure if she knew she was eating it. The day went on, the sleeves were added and the cookies were being consumed by all of us. When I went home I kept thinking about her trips to the cooling racks. As I was criticizing her in my mind, I realized that I ate an entire family size bag of Doritos! I was definitely a hypocrite but she was way worse off than me!

That's how I always judged things. I called it the Grading on the Manson Curve. I could be bad at something – doesn't matter what it is – as long as someone one is worse off then I feel better about it. In this example, I may have to lose a lot of weight BUT she has a lot more to lose SO I'm okay. By my own Manson Curve logic I could yell at someone and hurt their feelings BUT it's not like I'm Charles Manson! This is ridiculous but definitely a way that I looked at things. When I discovered that she had weight loss surgery in early 2002, I was surprised but not nearly as surprised as when I saw her.

It was serendipitous that I ran into her. I was stopping by a store that I never visit get things I never get and there she was. She said hello and it took me a second to register in my brain who it was. I know I tried to be casual but my face will often show what my brain is thinking without any help from me! I said hello and she only had a second to chat but I told her she looked great and she said thank you and that she hoped she'd see me again soon. As quickly as she popped up she was gone.

I was slightly shell-shocked. She looked amazing. To this very day, I can tell you what she was wearing because she had on one particular thing that heavy women generally try to avoid. She had on a double breasted peacoat completely buttoned! I couldn't believe it. That was a dream of mine: to wear a military style peacoat completely buttoned and to look amazing. She was living the dream. I was living the jealousy.

I couldn't stop thinking about her. Thinking that this was the same woman who couldn't pass a cooling rack! Weight loss surgery clearly performs miracles. I saw celebrity transformations but I also know that the rich and famous have access to far more things than we the common folk of the world. My friend was a common folk. She looked amazing. I started looking into weight loss surgery seriously on that day cold day in 2002. Unfortunately, I had a lot going on that year and much of it was pretty traumatic. Weight loss surgery was put on the backburner.

After the stairs in 2014, I took another look. I'd casually checked out different programs in the past for when I "got to that point." I still wasn't quite convinced I was there. I really should be able to do this on my own.

On Valentine's Day Eve I was going to bed with a touch of anxiety. Jeff is not an early riser and he's not a morning person. Every single day on Valentine's Day he wakes up early to place a card next to my sleeping face. It's really sweet to wake up to especially since it takes an extreme amount of effort for him to wake up early like that.

The next morning I woke to an amazing card. I should be happy. I should be grateful. I'm still just anxious. Why does he love me? When I lay on my back my neck feels like it's suffocating me. I can barely climb stairs and I sweat all the time. What does he see in me? This kind gesture provoked so many feelings that morning and not a single one of them good. I know he loves me. Why don't I love me? Why can't I love me? I was back on the internet before he even woke up for work. Weight loss surgery. Time to look again.

I came across an article written by a cardiologist that changed my life. He was writing about how so many people believe that weight loss surgery is drastic. I completely agreed with him. Weight loss surgery is definitely drastic. Then he wrote this:

Every single day I take a vein out of someone's leg and thread it through their heart and no one calls that drastic. That is drastic.

It was like bells and whistles went off in my head. For the first time, weight loss surgery wasn't a place where people went when they had no other option. It became a medical surgical procedure that can save lives. This one viewpoint changed everything for me. I went back and decided to look at surgery again but with this new perspective.

I was all in. I found a program that I liked that seemed to have a lot of support before and after surgery. Some places I looked at seemed very interested in getting people in surgery but not so much treating them or following up after. I decided it was time to tell Jeff that I was seriously considering weight loss surgery. He's my number one fan and the keenest supporter of every venture of mine.

"Jeff, I want to have weight loss surgery!" I exclaimed. I expected his usual kind and supportive answer. I did not get that.

"No!" he said way too quickly.

"Why not?" I asked.

"I love you just the way you are. Don't do that for me! People die doing that!"

The passion in his voice was almost overwhelming. It's not that he didn't want me to have surgery. He didn't want me to die. That was the day I had to share some truths with Jeff. It was hard to say it out loud but it had to be said.

"Jeff, as long as I'm alive like this I am staring death in the face. And, truth be told, I could leave this house and get hit by a bus so death is no longer an excuse for me not to do this."

He still wasn't convinced. I didn't have the heart to say out loud what I really needed to say. Jeff has always looked at me like I was the most beautiful woman in the room.

Always. I wanted to tell him that this surgery was for me. I wanted to love me the way he loves me. Even more, as a Christian, I wanted to love me the way He loves me. I just couldn't. I really wanted to. I just couldn't do it.

The program I chose had many requirements. The first was a consultation that went over the different types of procedures, the risk factors, how the program works, and many more details. I asked Jeff to go with me because I knew that he wasn't thrilled with this entire process but I really wanted him to see what it was about too.

We arrive at the hospital and there were about 25 people in the room. The nurse manager helmed the meeting with one of the surgeons. I was surprised to see that she not only ran the unit but she was a former patient. She had gastric bypass surgery nearly a decade before and she's done all kinds of running races since. I was encouraged that she kept the weight off.

As we went through the consult, I wasn't sure how to read Jeff. He was silently listening the entire time. After the nurse and surgeon went they had two people come up and share their experience in the program. The first was a police officer who was over 400 lbs and became a 200lb runner. The next was a woman who worked as a nurse and she had a pair of her old pants safety pinned to a pair of her new pants. I was blown away. These people had surgery only 2 years prior! Could that really be me?

When we left Jeff broke his silence. He took my hand and said the most beautiful thing to me. "I'm in. Whatever you want to do, I'm in. Surgery or no surgery, whatever you want I'm here to help."

I wondered what changed but I didn't ask. It was much later that he told me as the presentation was going on he was looking at the people around us. Many people were there alone. If they had a spouse the spouse wasn't there. If they didn't then they didn't even have a person to support them. He imagined them going through this process – that he didn't fully understand – all alone and he didn't like it. He also shared that he never saw in me what he saw around the room. He saw their sadness and the presentations showed him the dangers of obesity. He never considered me obese. He always considered me beautiful. Jeff has always loved my heart and not just what was wrapped around it.

We decided that we would go through this process like our marriage: together.

CHAPTER ELEVEN
FOOD FUNERALS

Many people aren't aware of the amount of time it takes from making the decision to have weight loss surgery to the actual surgery. After my consultation I was given a sheet of paper with 23 things that had to be accomplished before I could even approach my insurance company. Some of these items were medically necessary like having an upper GI and others were from the hospital like having 2 mandatory support group visits. All were to make sure that we were sufficiently prepared for surgery.

Every insurance company also has a list of requirements that you have to follow and it varies from plan to plan. My insurance company required 6 months of visits with a nutritionist unless you could prove you worked a medically supervised weight loss program in the past year. Lucky for me, I have six months of a failed medically supervised program on the books and that took the largest chunk of time from the process. I was getting more and more excited. I could feasibly be skinny by my birthday. What an amazing concept.

Another issue that takes up a bit of time is the scheduling of appointments. Trying to get appointments with Psychiatry and the Sleep Lab times was notoriously difficult. When I called to schedule my appointment with Psychiatry, I called on a Monday and had my appointment on Friday. I happened to call just as a person cancelled. Confirmation that Jesus also wanted me to have this surgery and be skinny by my birthday!

I was nervous about the psych appointment. I know two people who both failed the psych exam and were refused surgery. I was looking up what questions they would ask and how to answer them. Here I was – again – trying to game a system. I decided to just be honest with my answers and if I failed I would find out what I have to do to pass next time. I really want this to work.

The appointment was in two parts on the same day. I had to come in early and complete a written questionnaire. It took about an hour. Once that was done I had to return in the afternoon to speak with the doctor. She was a really nice woman and she asked me a lot of questions. I was very open with her. One thing that stands out from this appointment was her response when I told her I quit smoking 7 years earlier. She said that would give her the single greatest confidence that I would be successful at weight loss. I looked at her like she was crazy because my history would dictate otherwise.

She elaborated, "Smoking is a physical addiction as well as a social one and when you quit you are quitting more than simply smoking. You are quitting a social lifestyle as well as dealing with the physical withdrawals from smoking. You know how to miss something you craved. That will be instrumental here."

Wow! I never looked at quitting smoking like that. I never thought that my smoking and my eating were similar. I also never thought that I'd find a benefit from smoking. Looks like those eighteen years provided a little silver lining of hope. I passed psych with flying colors.

All of my other appointments were in quick succession. Things were going great. I was proving to be as "otherwise healthy" as my doctors would always say. This was a cause to celebrate and I know how to celebrate. I knew that once I was approved for surgery that there were certain foods that I'll never be able to have again. I set about to give them all a proper send off. Chocolate would be gone forever as will ice cream. I started eating them like they were going out of style because they really were for me.

I had food funerals everywhere! I was a permanent fixture at all buffets since I won't be able to enjoy a buffet again. My love of Ben and Jerry's was taken to an entirely new height. I had to give proper goodbyes. It was truly the only decent thing to do. I was gaining weight but I would worry about that when I got my surgical date. I wouldn't be able to even request it to my insurance company until after my sleep study which was proving hard to schedule.

Rhode Island is the smallest state and we act like our state is the size of Texas! Many of us from southern RI don't like to travel too far north if we don't have to. My surgical program was about 40 miles north and I was doing a fair amount of driving back and forth.

It was driving me crazy. When I went to finally schedule my sleep study I couldn't get an appointment at the recommended place for several months. Everything was going so smoothly and here was a bump in the road. I called the program office and asked if I could possibly go to a different place, perhaps one closer to where I live. They said that was fine so I booked my appointment at the hospital down the road from my house. They could fit me in within five days. We are back on schedule!

I didn't think much of the sleep study. I really thought sleep apnea was not a big deal and I didn't understand why we had to do it but it was required so I did it.

I arrived at the hospital at 10pm and entered what looked like an abandoned area of the hospital. The sleep lab is very quiet and very private. The lab technician was really nice and got me all hooked up. I looked like a crazy person. I had no idea how I was ever going to sleep with all these wires everywhere. I don't sleep well normally so this would be interesting.

The lab looked like a bedroom and I appreciated that they tried really hard to not make it seem as normal an experience as possible. If it were a standard hospital room I would have never fallen asleep.

I watched television for a while and then read a little bit trying to think of the person on the other side of the glass that's clearly waiting for me to fall asleep. It seemed like it took a long time but I finally fell asleep.

Next thing I know, the attendant is waking me. I'm startled and disoriented. I had to take a second to remember where I was.

"Mrs. Bartlett, I'm going to put the mask on you now," he said. He placed the nasal pillow mask on my face and I went back to sleep.

The next morning was interesting. The attendant said I did fine and I asked what the verdict was. He said that he administers the test but a respiratory therapist will read the results and contact me. I was still not thinking sleep apnea was a big deal. That quickly changed.

I got the call to see the respiratory therapist at the surgical supply place that afternoon. I don't recall any test getting any type of result that quickly. I walk in and he's very pleasant and offers me a seat.

"Mrs. Bartlett, can you please hold your

breath?" he asks.

"What?" I question.

"Can you please hold your breath. Just hold it in for as long as you can and I'll time you."

"Okay..." I'm instantly suspect but I hold my breath.

It's not very comfortable for me to hold my breath. I held it for a short time and just ended the madness. I wanted to know what his point was here.

"Twelve seconds," He said. "Do you know how long you held your breath during your sleep study?"

"No," I answered but definitely curious.

"Sixty-four seconds. You went over a minute without breathing and that was just the longest time. You stopped breathing hundreds of time during the study. He woke you up to put the mask on you because it was too dangerous to continue to test. I'd be willing to bet you haven't had a solid night's rest in years!"

I didn't even know how to respond! I was stunned that I held my breath for over a minute at one time let alone that I continuously stopped breathing.

He went on to tell me about the dangers of sleep apnea. How each time you stop breathing your body is deprived of air which will begin to break down your organs over time. He also let me know that chronic sleep apnea is most likely responsible for car accidents and other related events since people are unwittingly exhausted from not getting decent sleep.

I was fitted with a CPAP machine and went home with a whole new understanding of sleep apnea. You could really die from sleep apnea and now I understand why it was so important to have this test done. I was also requited to bring my CPAP to the hospital for surgery if I was approved.

Even with the small nasal pillow mask it was an adjustment using the machine. The first few days felt like the air was trying to blow out my eardrums. After the initial discomfort it was wonderful. I would wake up feeling relaxed and refreshed which I never thought I'd feel upon waking.

I shared a lot of my experience on

Facebook because there were so many people who felt like I did thinking that sleep apnea was a throw away condition. It can be serious and even fatal. I counted my blessings that I was tested and treated.

I completed my sleep study just after the Fourth of July. It was the last item I had to cross of my list before the hospital could submit to my insurance company for approval. As I waited my food funerals were getting more and more extensive and my weight gain was adding up. I thought about slowing down my food consumption but then I thought if I was denied surgery it would all be for nothing so I continued to eat.

I lost a lot of time scheduling my sleep study. My plan to be skinny by my birthday seemed unlikely at best. Smaller, maybe, but definitely not skinny. I was pretty upset by that. At the beginning of this process it looked like God was taking the reins and moving mountains and now I'm out here alone – still fat – with no idea when or even IF I'll be able to have surgery. The food funerals continued.

I finally got the notification that my insurance company approved my surgery and I was able to take the final steps to surgery. I realized that I gained a lot of weight and I had to address that immediately. There's a lot of talk on internet forums about how some hospitals will cancel your surgery if you gain weight during pre-operative testing. I whittled my food way back and did away with the funerals. I couldn't see my doctor again with weight gain. She hadn't seen me in months and the last thing I wanted to be was drastically overweight from before.

The final piece to my pre-op puzzle arrived in August 2014, I had to have an h. pylori test completed. I didn't even know what it was and I didn't care. It was the last hurdle. I was going through the last flaming hoop before surgery. It's August and maybe I'll have surgery by my birthday instead of being skinny for my birthday. I'll accept that!

When I went to the testing facility the technician was a little unsure about the test. She knew I had to drink something awful but she admitted she wasn't too familiar with the test. I wasn't concerned. We did it and it seemed fine.

Two weeks later and two weeks before my birthday, my doctor called to tell me that the test was improperly administered. I asked her to tell me what that means for my surgery. She explained that I have to retake the test but I have to wait two weeks before I retest and if I'm positive for h. pylori then I have to be treated with antibiotics for a month and then retake the test again.

WHAT? Now, I'm well beyond my birthday! This is crazy. I asked if I could just be treated now like I have it – whatever it is – and then retest to see if I'm negative. Apparently, it doesn't work like that. I would have to wait anywhere from 5-9 weeks before I could have surgery. At this point I'm also getting close to the end of the year where my deductible will reset and I'll have to pay a lot of money out of pocket for surgery. This was the worst news. I couldn't be more upset after this phone call. I was wrong.

I went for my retest and I retested as positive for h. pylori so now I had to be treated with antibiotics and retest. I was definitely more upset than I was before.

Looking back, I'm glad they test and retest because they discovered that the bacteria h. pylori is present is most cases of stomach cancer and cutting into my stomach with this active bacteria wouldn't be a good thing at all. I can see that clearly now. Then I only saw yet another road block on my way to being skinny by my birthday. Maybe God I telling me that I shouldn't do this. That's got to be it because why else would this be happening.

I turned 42 years old on September 8, 2014. I was crammed into the booth at a chain restaurant. They had no tables available so my husband and mom sat on one side and I took up the entire other side. I was so uncomfortable.

After dinner they surprised me with birthday cake. This would be the final food funeral. After we sang my mother told me to make a wish.

I remember how excited I was that I was finally taking the steps to surgery in March. I remember sailing through the pre-op process in the beginning. I remember desperately wanting to be skinny by this day. Here I am still big and looking for wishes. I was all wished out. I decided to pray. I closed my eyes and I did something I have never done. I called upon the Lord directly about my weight. I asked God to take it. My weight has always been my problem. Something I tried to fix. I failed every single time but it was always my issue.

No one else's. Not even God's and that had to change.

In that moment, with my eyes closed my heart cried out to Him that it's entirely in His hands. When or if I have surgery, how the outcome would be, everything was His. It's been tight-fisted in my hands for 30 years and today it belongs only to Him.

I blew out the candle and I was immediately washed in peace. I could hear God whisper in my ear that this was all He ever wanted from me. I had to surrender completely. I wasn't skinny by my birthday, but I was completely free.

Everything seemed to go at warp speed from that moment. My h. pylori was treated and cleared and my last pre-op appointment was scheduled for October. If all goes well, I can make the calendar by December and stay in the same insurance benefit year. I didn't stress, I left it all to God.

On the morning of my appointment I was concerned about my weight. Although I didn't step on the scale since my last appointment before the food funerals I knew I had lost a good amount of weight leading up to this day. I was just hoping to be around the same. I didn't have to lose anything but I didn't want to gain anything. Everything was perfect and I was scheduled for December 10, 2014.

Thanksgiving. One would think that it would be the ultimate food funeral. I was actually fine at Thanksgiving. I didn't eat too much or go too far. I had my eye on the prize. So many family members questioned why I would have surgery so close to Christmas. The consensus was that I should wait until after the holiday.

Here's my thought on that topic. I wait until after Christmas then it's New Year's Eve, then it's Valentine's Day, then it's St. Patrick's Day and then and then and then. There's always something! If it's not a federal holiday that centers around food and drink then it's someone's birthday. There will always be a reason to celebrate. Always. Not to mention that doing it in the same benefit year is financially better.

Just after Thanksgiving the surgeon's office called and asked if I wanted to push my surgery ahead to December 3rd. They had a patient scheduled that day that had a conflict and asked if I would mind switching. I was thrilled.

One thing I noticed from my birthday to that day was than when I fully surrendered my weight to God I no longer carried any burden with it. My anxiety about this process and my expectations about it were gone. I left it to Him and He showed me that was where it belonged all along.

Cast all your anxiety on Him because He cares for you." 1 Peter 5:7 NIV

CHAPTER TWELVE
SURGERY DAY & TOO MUCH TIME

The night before surgery I had to take a special shower with some special soap to prevent infections and affix an anti-nausea patch behind my ear. It was finally happening. I've thought about this since the dawn of Carnie Wilson and it was finally happening.

My surgery was scheduled at 11am but I had to report to the hospital for 8am. Jeff and I made the trip mostly in silence. We both had our concerns that I think we were too afraid to share. Death is a complication of every surgery. Although rare it is possible. I know we were both feeling that reality.

In the parking lot he took my hand and kissed it then placed it in his lap.

"Father God, please place a special anointing on Regina today with her surgery. Guide the hands of her surgeon and team and let Your will be done. Everything that happens is for Your glory. Amen."

Again, there was a wash of peace over me as we walked into the hospital. We stayed together as long as we could and then we finally had to part. I was comfortable and ready.

The next thing I remember is someone yelling at me to walk. Everything around me was blurry and it seemed like it was going in super-fast motion.

The next time I open my eyes I'm in a hospital bed in a private room. I see my glasses, cellphone, and iPad on the stand next to me. I put on my glasses and look at the clock. It's 10pm! What happened?

Apparently, I was out like a light for hours. The nurses had me walk when I was in the recovery room and then I was transferred upstairs to my room. Jeff stayed with me for hours but finally had to leave to take care of the dogs. He sent me the sweetest text messages.

A nurse comes in an immediately calls me Sleeping Beauty. After a while they were going to have to force me awake if I didn't wake up on my own. She told me to rest up because tomorrow the work begins.

I woke up early the next morning. I was asked to take a quick walk around the floor and return for breakfast. I wasn't sure how I was going to feel. I didn't have any discomfort at all. If I didn't have tape over my incisions I wouldn't have believed I had surgery. I felt fine, but I knew that the drugs would eventually wear off.

I got out of the bed and I was surprised at how well I could walk. I went past the other rooms and some people didn't want to walk, others had pain, and here I was walking pain free. Thank you, Jesus!

I made my way back to my room to find my "breakfast" was delivered. It was a protein shake and a little measuring cup to portion it. I was to drink about ½ ounce at a time. It was at this time that I knew that I really did have surgery. Sipping that took forever! By the time I was done with one ounce several hours had gone by and "lunch" was being delivered.

Jeff arrived and it was so good to see him. He kept apologizing for leaving before I woke up. I was grateful to have a partner that knows that the puppies require consistency and it was just as important for him to be home as it was for him to be here with me. He already talked to the surgeon before he left and knew that I was recovering well. I showed him my breakfast and lunch. At this rate I will be taking home 2 days of protein shakes at discharge!

Jeff stayed the day with me and went walking and gave me encouragements to drink the shakes. Not moments after he left two of my friends came in! I was surprised to see them because Rhode Islanders being what we are with driving I never expected them to come up to Providence to see me. I was so grateful.

It was during their visit that I got my second clue about my surgery. Physically, I was fine but drinking the shakes was the first clue that my body was definitely different. The second one was laughter.

I think I nearly busted two stiches when then came in! I was blessed to have my husband be so supportive but my friends making the trip was unbelievably special. Even if I thought I may need another surgery after they left. I was going to be okay. I knew it.

When I was released home I felt really prepared. The hospital was very detailed on what to expect, what do to, what not to do through each dietary phase. I was going to be on pureed foods for a few weeks, but I had a lot of instructions on how to make that work.

One of the questions that I get asked the most is about this time frame. How much time did you take off of work after surgery? This is going to be dependent on the work you do and I was not working at the time. What I will say is that you will need the amount of time necessary to get your new life in order. You have to find a rhythm to this new way of living. Getting in enough water, eating the right things at the right time, getting in enough protein, and taking your vitamins are all essential. There are even some vitamins that can't be taken at the same time so you have to be sure that you're spacing everything properly. People are hospitalized after surgery most often for dehydration. I was grateful that I didn't have the pressure to return to work while I took the time to really figure this part out.

The hardest part of the first ten days after surgery was the shots. I had to give myself a shot in the stomach twice a day for ten days. It was a blood thinner to prevent blood clots. Blood clots can be fatal and after surgery they are focused on making sure you keep your blood moving by walking and taking the shots.

Jeff is a Type 1 Diabetic and for years I've watched him take shots in his belly five times a day. I remember helping my grandfather by giving him insulin shots in his thigh. I never once thought of how emotionally draining that can be. The shots were the worst but before I could take a moment and feel sorry for myself I just thought of Jeff and how he's taken about 30,000 shots since his diagnosis. I really can't complain at all.

Jeff works a lot and I hadn't been working since the start-up company was sold. I was used to being at home. What I wasn't used to was the amount of time.

I was a volume eater. I could eat a lot in a single sitting. If I wasn't actively eating, I was planning my next meal, cooking it, or thinking about it. Food was always on my mind. On those first days after surgery I found myself with an unprecedented amount of time on my hands. Which was funny because before it seemed like I could never get anything done!

I distinctly remember the day Jeff came home and I nearly attacked him when he came in.

"I need a job!" I exclaimed.

"You just had surgery, you can't work right now," he said.

"I know that but as soon as I'm able I have to work. This is madness. I have so much time on my hands! I never knew just how much space in my life was dedicated to eating until I was no longer eating!"

I think he was afraid of me in that moment. I don't blame him, I was scary excited, nervous, and fresh from surgery with a sudden realization that I spent most days in search of food.

I was already planning to be very open about surgery because when I was seriously considering this a few months back I couldn't find anyone that had the surgery. I wanted a first-hand account. The internet has a lot of information but you never know what's real online. It's like 1 part fact and 9 parts garbage and you never really know what's what.

I've blogged throughout my life. Since the birth of the internet in mass use. I decided to blog again and really focus on this process. I also kept a journal to remind of feelings in the moment. That took up some of my time. That was good. Writing can be very exhausting emotional work. After which I have to settle my brain by watching something pointless on television.

Sitting for long periods of time isn't good. I was required to walk but I wasn't comfortable going outside. I decided to Earn My TV. When I wanted to watch television I had to take steps in front of the TV while my show was on. Once a commercial came on I could take a break, get a glass or water, or take a seat. As soon as my show came back on then I came back on! I started gaining some steps each day and it was getting easier and easier to walk. I decided it was time to venture outside.

Having a dog makes it easy to go on walks. I decided to take my little whippersnapper nugget Sid Vicious out for a walk. This tiny yet mighty Chihuahua gets a bulk of his walking on the long yard lead that lets him own our backyard. I decided to bundle the little guy up and take him on the street. Where we live is very desolate in winter so there's hardly anyone on the road.

Not five seconds into our first walk and I noticed that something changed in our little pup. He loved it. He was smelling everything and wanting to explore everywhere. There's a private road across the street that has a little pond and made it there and decided to turn around. I wasn't sure how far his tiny legs would take him. When I got home I went online and looked at maps of our neighborhood. I decided to make some goals for both of us. We already made it to the pond. There's another large body of water through the neighborhood after the little pond. That will be our next goal. Each day we set another plan and Sid Vicious was in love with walking. Some days I found it hard to keep up with him!

The first pond was half mile away. The large pond was three quarter miles away. The ocean was a full mile from our doorstep to toes in the sand. It was getting easier every day for both of us. Every morning we wake up and go out. It got to the point where as soon as I opened my eyes he was jumping in front of the leash. He didn't just want to go outside he wanted to explore.

This time was more than time spent with my dog. This was time in reflective prayer. Every day I would marvel at the beauty around me. God is so present during the predawn hour walks. You get to see and experience a peace that makes you pause and just be grateful.

After 4 months I got a job at a local dentist office that was close to my house. It was nice to be out and about again. I was down almost 100lbs and I would walk two to five miles in the morning before work.

One day at closing time I was making sure there was toilet paper and paper towels in the patient bathroom and I caught my reflection in the mirror. I had collarbones! I don't think I've ever had visible collar bones in my life. I went home and I couldn't wait to tell Jeff about my newly visible bones.

He was very happy for me but he had a weird look about him. He told me that it's time for me to get new pants. My pants looked really big. I wasn't ready for pants. I certainly didn't want to buy pants only to buy more pants in a few weeks. I could let these pants work for a few more weeks.

A couple of weeks later I was in the downstairs office alone. Thank goodness. I got up from my chair and went to walk into the hall and my pants hit the floor. The floor. I was standing in the hallway with my pants around my ankles and my underwear in clear view of the earth. No one was in the hall – which is a bit of a miracle because it's a very busy dentist office. After my initial shock I scrambled to pull my pants up and immediately went back to my desk. Mark it on the calendar. My husband was right, it was time for new pants.

I wasn't going to tell him about my big underwear reveal at work since no one saw it. If a staff member loses her pants in the hall and no one was there to see it, did it really happen? No. That answer is no.

After Jeff and I had dinner I was getting up to go into the kitchen. He asked if I could bring something in the kitchen for him. To this day, I don't remember what I was carrying but I know it required both of my hands. As I was walking into the kitchen my pants fell again and I nearly tripped and fell. I looked like a buffoon because Jeff was laughing hysterically.

I put the item I was carrying down and I put my pants back on. I stepped out of one of the legs completely trying not to drop my cargo. Once I get my pants back on I take one step and it was very uncomfortable. I wasn't sure what was happening. Then I realized what I did and walked back into the living room.

I just stare at Jeff. He doesn't understand why I'm just standing there looking at him. Then he finally realizes what happened. In my hurry to put my pants back on for the second time that day I put both of my legs in ONE leg of my pants. It was officially time to get new pants when you can fit both of your legs in one side. We went directly to the store... laughing all the way.

CHAPTER THIRTEEN
HOT AND READY CAR RIDE

Food was always more than food to me. It was my comforter, my boyfriend that I dated exclusively for years, and it was the main way that I handled disappointment, fear, or anxiety. Food was everything. Those first few protective months after surgery is almost womb like. Everyone knew that I was having surgery because it was my choice to tell them. I've always been proven to be way too untrustworthy with food. I needed all the accountability partners I could rustle up!

When things became stressful in my life, a little apple pie could always take edge off a bad day. When you no longer have food as you primary problem solver, you are at a disadvantage. I was a person that was filled with silent rage. I would rarely vocalize how I was feeling. Instead, I would swallow my feelings usually with ice cream and then move on. Not the most advantageous way of handling issues but it "worked" for me for thirty years.

My job was stressful. It was a very busy practice with a lot of moving pieces and a lot of people to please. Now, my stress had nowhere to go. My morning walks were turning into morning runs and mini prayer services and that definitely helped. One day everything changed.

Jeff and I took two of our grandkids overnight so their parents could go away. They really good kids but very active. It's hard having little kids around especially after not having them in so long. We discovered our house was woefully not child proof and our puppy didn't like playing second fiddle to the grandkids. It was a stressful day.

The next day our original plan was to take the kids to church with us but we saw that it would be hard for them to sit still that long and since they weren't familiar with anyone at church it could be challenging for them if we tried to put them in the nursery. We finally decided that I would drop Jeff off at church and I would bring the kids home.

All the way to their house my grandson

kicked the back of my chair. I asked several times to stop but he continued. I know he just wanted to go home after spending a night of hearing "No, don't touch that" was just as hard for him as it was for us. Neither child slept well that night either. They both just wanted their parents. I wanted them pretty badly too.

The kids had moved not too long before this day and I had only been to their house once before. In true form of a person in their 40s who still believes they remember things, I thought I knew where I was going. I pull into the driveway of their apartment and my grandson says "This is not my house." I was sure it was. He was sure it wasn't. Granted he was only 5 years old but it was where he lived I should've believed him.

I call the parents and tell them I'm outside. They aren't home yet. The kicks will continue on the back of my seat for another 40 minutes while they wait for the bus. I decide to ask them their house number and sure enough, 5 year old definitely know where they live. Both kids don't want to wait in the car they want to go to their house. I decide to go to the store to pick up their parents so they don't have to wait for the bus. I was never so happy to drive a three row van in my life.

After 40 miles, almost non-stop kicking on the back of my seat, intermittent tears, and parental rescue, and reaching the correct house I was on my way home. I missed the on ramp for the highway and had to go through town for a bit. Then I saw it. Like a beacon in the sky the Little Caesar's sign was glowing HOT & READY. An entire pizza for $5. That sounds amazing. My mouth was watering. Pizza could fix these feelings. Fast! I even had a $5 bill in my car! I could get this pizza and no one would know.

Before I realized what was happening I was in the line ordering a $5 pizza. It would be ready in a minute. As I stood there in line I started thinking of my life. Food was always my answer no matter the question. Look where that's got me. I'm down over 150 lbs. and I walk every day and I'm getting things done. Why am I in here?

Cash. I came in here because I had cash. I remember when Jeff and I joined our accounts. I remember being really resentful because I could no longer eat at my leisure. I had someone else to look over my spending and he would be horrified if he saw exactly how much I was eating.

I remember finding safe zones to buy food. These are places that I could safely buy food without fear or judgement. Craft stores always have sweets and dollar stores always have all kinds of food. Since I would normally shop at these places it wasn't unusual to see purchases there. If I went to fast food places 3 times a day and then came home to eat dinner then that would be a cause for questions.

I already ordered the food on a whim looking to release my feelings of my trip. I had surgery 6 months ago and I don't even know what my body would do if I ate this pizza! What was I thinking. As the worker starts to cut and box my fresh from the oven pizza an older, overweight man walks in the store. He seems tired and just ordered food like I would order food. I used to order like I was ordering for a ton of people when I knew it was just for me. I've been known to order 4 drinks so it looked like 4 people would be eating with me. I fooled no one, I'm sure, but myself. What am I doing here? I took the pizza and put it in the car. The smell was amazing. The very smell made me feel better.

Dumping syndrome is a very real thing with RNY Gastric Bypass surgery. What you're bypassing in RNY Gastric Bypass surgery is the small intestines so the food you eat goes you're your new smaller stomach pouch and then directly into your large intestines. The large intestines don't process sugar or fat well the small intestines usually cover that job. After RNY Gastric Bypass, if you eat too much sugar or fat you can have a reaction called dumping syndrome. Dumping syndrome doesn't affect people in the same ways and it doesn't affect some people at all. Some people will vomit immediately, others may poop quickly and without warning, and still others may get sweats and shakes. The worst thing for me would be to not get anything at all. I needed my internal accountability partner just as much as my external ones.

Being 6 months out of surgery I wasn't about to eat the pizza. I did, however, keep it on the front seat and smelled it until my highway exit where I went through a coffee shop drive through and pitched it in the trash. I don't like to waste food but I also didn't want any evidence.

As I pulled into the church God made it clear to me that I was supposed to reach out to Him in my time of stress not pizza. Not surprisingly, I opened my bible directly to:

11 In the same way, count yourselves dead to sin but alive to God in Christ Jesus.12 Therefore do not let sin reign in your mortal body so that you obey its

*evil desires. 13 Do not offer any part of yourself to
sin as an instrument of wickedness, but rather offer
yourselves to God as those who have been brought
from death to life; and offer every part of yourself to
him as an instrument of righteousness.14 For sin
shall no longer be your master, because you are not
under the law, but under grace.*
Romans 6:11-14 NIV

I was kindly reminded that I needed to fall on my knees and not fall into a pizza shop when my feelings became more than I could handle.

CHAPTER FOURTEEN
ELBOWING IN THE KITCHEN

I was never much of a cook. Ask anyone. One time on social media my son was playing one of those social interview games where it would ask you randomly selected questions about people on your friend's list. He got this one: How has your life improved since you met Jeff Bartlett? His answer: I no longer have to eat my mother's cooking. That makes it pretty clear that my cooking left a lot to be desired.

Jeff loves to cook and he loves to cook for people. The more the merrier. We would always have family or friends over and Jeff would prepare these elaborate meals. Thanksgiving was always his favorite holiday and he would pull out all the stops to make the most wonderful tasting and memorable meals.

As I started to reintroduce food into my diet I noticed that Jeff would cook something for me and then something for him. I know he likes to cook but it made me feel like I was a separate person and meals are to be shared.

We could both have cod. But Jeff likes his cod with butter and crackers, and I couldn't have it that way. He'd poach or steam mine and then cook his. I was learning a lot about my new way of eating. The most important thing was that there was a lot of unnecessary fat and sugar in the way that we were cooking. Food was tasting just fine without an entire dump truck of butter. Jeff was convinced I thought things tasted okay because I haven't had it in any other way in so long that my taste buds were shot. I formulated a plan.

I've been reading all kinds of books on healthy cooking and I was eager to try some recipes and even try to make some of my favorite recipes still taste good without compromising my goals. The first one I wanted to try was zucchini "pasta." I ordered a spiralizer from Amazon and went to work.

Jeff had zero interest in my fake pasta. He was going to cook something else but thought it was cute that I was going to try cooking. Cooking was officially something where I was rarely successful unless you count my amazing shepherd's pie that Jeff ultimately made better.

I went to work spiralizing the noodles and it was really easy to do. In a pan I took 90% lean ground beef and browned it. After I drained the beef I added fresh tomatoes and spices and let it cook together. The smell was wonderful and began to waft into the living room where the unsuspecting Jeff was curious.

"What are you cooking?" he asked.

"Just something for me, used my spiralizer!"

"That smells really good. Can I taste it?"

I almost passed out! He wanted to taste my food? MY food? That I cooked? The planets must be aligned for this event to be happening. I tried to play it cool.

"Oh, I thought you wanted something else," I tried to not sound like I was excited although I was quite exited he wanted some.

"Well, maybe I can try a little," he said.

I took my sauce mixture and added the zucchini noodles and cooked them together. I plated it for both of us and we sat down for dinner.

At first he was a little suspect about how it would taste since I have a history of not being the best cook. The look in his eyes after the first bite was all I needed to know about how it tasted. He loved it.

That first day gave me all the confidence I needed to continue in the kitchen. I started with items I was comfortable cooking. In time, I moved on to thinking of foods I used to love but would no longer work after RNY Gastric Bypass. It became a challenge that I savored. Can I make this look and taste good for both of us?

My goal was to make sure that we could eat together. I was fine if he wanted to make something occasionally that wasn't suitable for me. I just wanted to be sure that we didn't live completely separate dietary lives.

Jeff was so into the recipes I was trying and the foods that I was altering to make them bariatric friendly that he joined me in the kitchen. Together we have worked on many dishes that not only taste flavorful but are also healthy.

Our friends were also quick to realize that Jeff was looking heathier every time they saw him too. It's called the Halo Effect when one person in a family decides to get healthier and it radiates to others.

Sausage stuffed onions, Italian Zucchini Boats, Cucumber Grinders and No Muffin Banana Muffins were big hits at social events. After the success of my No Muffin Banana Muffins I took to baking and working to mimic something healthy that also gave the feel of something decadent.

Every time I ate in public people would ask me about what I can't and can eat. I understand their curiosity. There are so many questions and misunderstandings about weight loss surgery. It was pleasure to share what I was eating. One evening I even invited my friends over for dinner to showcase that even without weight loss surgery, you can eat well and be satisfied. They were pleasantly surprised at the taste of the food. My portion was a little shocking for them but the food was great.

Since that dinner I've been working on a cookbook of fully original recipes. I published a small eBook teaser of recipes that was well received. I knew I was on to something.

One of the great barriers with people considering surgery is that they fear they won't be able to enjoy food. You can enjoy food but it's essential to change your relationship with food. For many people food isn't just food. It's comfort, hope, peace, and joy and if you can't reach those feelings without using food then that's where you have to work before surgery or anything else will work for you.

Another barrier is that people don't want to feel restricted. They think that after weight loss surgery our stringent dietary needs are a problem. Limiting sugar, fat, and carbs can seem pretty daunting as is eliminating junk food and fast foods from your diet. I know I didn't think I could do it at first!

Over time things change. Your perspective shifts and so do your priorities. Now, what seems restrictive to some is just life to me. It isn't a diet as much as it's simply a typical day in my world. It becomes second nature almost like it was always there. You can develop a new instinct.

There is life after cake, there is joy in zucchini, and a simple perspective shift can make a huge difference in your long term success. The goal is to strive to make your "can't haves" into your "don't wants." I do this, one new recipe at a time. Here's one to try at home.

Italian Zucchini Boats

4 zucchini
1 lb. lean ground beef
Italian Seasoning
1 cup diced tomato
Mozzarella cheese
Preheat oven to 350

In skillet brown ground beef and take one of the zucchini and dice it and add to meat. Add tomatoes and season to taste.

Take remaining 3 zucchini and cut off ends and cut lengthwise. Scoop out centers to form boat and place on glass baking sheet with nonstick cooking spray.

Spoon meat mixture into boats and top with Mozzarella. Bake at 350 for 15 min.

CHAPTER FIFTEEN
THE BEAUTY OF BEING SEEN

Envy. Such a bitter place to be yet I spent a ton of time there. I'd always look at movie stars, athletes, even fit people next to me at the grocery store; all with equal envy. I wanted that body. I wanted to feel that good about myself. I wanted to wear those clothes. I wanted what they had. It all seemed so unattainable to me. Instead doing something to advance those desires, I would sit on the couch eating Ben & Jerry's by the pint and be envious of all they had and all they were able to do. I can't imagine how much time I wasted doing that. Dreaming of a life while sitting down and almost guaranteeing it would never happen for me.

I remember when Oprah Winfrey lugged that red wagon out on her show with the representation of 80lbs of fat that she lost on her first public diet. I also remember thinking that if I had millions of dollars, a personal chef, and virtually unlimited funds that I, too, could truck out a wagon of fat. I love Oprah but this didn't motivate me at all. If anything, it only fueled my envy. Again, unattainable. Cue the Ben & Jerry's!

Then Oprah did something that really opened my eyes. She ran a marathon. Why was this a game changer? Here's what her trainer Bob Greene said in an interview (paraphrased):

People give Oprah zero respect with her weight loss because she's rich and she as access to personal chefs and home gyms but what they don't understand is that to run a marathon you have to train. Her chef isn't getting up at 4am to run 10 miles before a full day of filming. She's doing that. She works more hours than most people can imagine and she puts in the time to do this. No one can run a marathon for you. You have to do it yourself and she is doing it.

And she really did it. She completed the Chicago marathon in 4:34! Impressive for a first time marathoner. What she also did was show the world that things can be done. She put the marathon into an accessible category for people who are not marathoners. Like me. I was always fascinated by distance runners but never thought I could be one. Marathon running became this check box on a distant bucket list that will never ticked to completion. I just stayed envious of those who completed them.

What became very apparent with weight loss surgery was the level of desire to succeed you have to have to make a long term change. That's what I'd been missing all along. The dream is free but the hustle costs extra. I never had the hustle but I lived in dreams. That's what made the difference with Oprah running the marathon. She could want it but if she didn't put in the work she wouldn't get there.

From that day in 1994, I wanted to run a marathon too. I did the Hyannis Half Marathon in 2008, coming in dead last but crossing the finish line. I vowed to go back and finish it. Then life happens.

Now, it's late 2015, and I'm putting in some serious miles every day. When you spend so much time out in nature with nothing but your thoughts in rhythm with your playlist, your mind goes to crazy places. Marathon places. Should I do it? Should I go back to Hyannis like I always said I would? Reality quickly returns when you realize that the Hyannis Marathon is in February and only 60 days away. That's not nearly enough time to train. I kept moving and kept thinking.

By the time February 2016, came around I was all but decided that I was going to run a marathon. I needed enough time to train so it had to be at least a 6 months away. I posed the question to my friends on Facebook to see if anyone was planning a late year Marathon. One of my friends who was living in Minnesota was planning on doing the NYC Marathon in November. She was using her race entry from 2012 when they didn't have the marathon because of Super Storm Sandy. I decided to take her up on running the NYC Marathon as a charity runner. I had to register right away before I thought better of it and changed my mind.

Running for cancer awareness was just the motivation I needed to take this challenge on full force. After losing my cousin Sybil,

what better way to honor her memory. I
started to think of so many other people in
my life who have been affected by cancer's
grasp. No family has been immune to cancer.
I decided to reach out to my childhood best
friend who lost her mom to cancer to ask her
if she minded if I ran in her mom's honor.
She then told me that she was diagnosed with
breast cancer so I could run for her too. I
became a woman on a mission after that. One
of the kindest and most influential people of
my life whose very presence shaped and
molded so much was diagnosed with breast
cancer. It seemed like only yesterday we were
carefree teenagers driving around the beaches
of Westerly with not a single care in the
world. I owe her so much in my life that I
needed to do this even more than before.

To do it, I know I have to do it right! One
thing I learned from the half marathon is that
the proper shoe is essential in long distance
running. Each shoe is designed with different
features and every person has unique features
that make some shoes better than others. It
took me 45 minutes at a specialty running
store to find the right shoe. Since most long
distance runners are generally small, finding a
shoe with a sturdier base and overall support
was going to be important. I found the

perfect shoe and then set the next task of planning my training schedule.

Marathon training plans are very detailed, especially for new runners. You generally run three times a week in increasing distances with one long run at the end of the week. Running three times a week in the beginning is fine. Your distances start out like 3 miles, 4 miles, 6 miles. I would run on Tuesdays, Thursdays, and Sundays. Those shorter runs are easy to accomplish before or after work so I was able to sail through the first few weeks.

Each week the mileage increases a little so you're eased into longer distances. As time went on it was getting harder and harder to run before work. Doing 6 miles in the morning then working a 10 hour day was a challenge. It was equally challenging to work a 10 hour day and then run 6 miles.

I'll never forget the day that I worked all day and then banged out a quick 8 miles. I was running on the bike path in the next town because it was open, had mile markers, and very few areas that cross traffic so I could really focus on what I was doing without fearing cars. As I was getting back into my car to drive home it hit me that I just worked an entire day and THEN ran 8 miles. This is the same woman who could barely climb a flight of stairs just over a year ago.

Weight loss surgery has so many misconceptions. Many people believe that this process is taking the easy way out. Others wonder why people just don't eat well or have any willpower. They just don't understand this process.

On a very hot long run Sunday I just completed 11 miles. I was covered in sweat and exhausted. I stopped by the store on my way home and ran into a person I hadn't seen in decades. I knew the reaction I would receive. I was easily 150lbs lighter than when she saw me last and it showed on her face.

"Regina! Oh my goodness you look amazing. What are you doing?" she asked.

"Well, I had RNY Gastric Bypass and I started runn…" In mid-sentence she cut me off.

"Oh, darn. Surgery. I was really hoping you worked for it," with the sound of condescension dripping from her lips.

At first I felt like I was punched in the face. Then it quickly morphed to anger. I may have had surgery but it didn't surgically remove my love of ice cream and surgery didn't just run 11 miles! I had to pause and take a step back because I remember that I was there too. I was the person who thought weight loss surgery was the easy way out. I just smiled and walked away.

Fools give full vent to their rage, but the wise bring calm in the end. Proverbs 29:11 NIV

When I got back to my car I cried for a few minutes. I can't let these things bother me. No one will understand if no one tells them. God hears even the unspoken prayers. I got a notification on my phone. It was a picture on my Facebook wall from one of my friend Jaime. God used her to answer the call from my heart.

The picture was titled The Iceberg Illusion and it reads SUCCESS IS AN ICEBERG. The top of the iceberg is what everyone sees: SUCCESS! Below the water was the largest, unseen part of the iceberg and it showed what most people don't see: failure, determination, discipline, and work.

She was letting me know that she sees me. She sees the work that I'm putting in and she understands that it's not all sunshine and roses. This was actually the second time she blessed me with seeing my effort. She called me on the phone one day to tell me that she drives by my workplace often and when she does she notices that I always park at the far end of the lot. She can see that I was trying to get my steps in and taking every opportunity to work and she notices it. I was so blessed by her picture and it gave me the strength to continue running and to remember that God always hears, always listens, and always understands.

CHAPTER SIXTEEN
THE SUMMER OF LIVING

I spent the entire summer of 2016, working and running. Jeff bought me a shirt from a Christian athletic apparel company with my favorite verse:

Those who wait on the Lord
Shall renew their strength;
They shall mount up with wings like eagles,
They shall run and not be weary,
They shall walk and not faint. Isaiah 40:31 NIV

There were a lot of organizational changes that happened at work and I just didn't feel connected. I decided to give my notice. I spent many years living a sedentary life. I let opportunities pass me by waiting for the time I felt I was ready. If I lose (enter amount of weight here) then I'll (enter whatever dream I want here). So much time waiting. So much time being unhappy. Now, I'm an active participant at life. I run nearly every day, I eat well, and my mind is clearer than it had been in ages. Why would I want to stay anywhere that wasn't bringing me absolute joy? One day Jeff said this to me: Do you know what I miss? My happy wife.

A week after my last day of work, one hundred seven members of my family boarded a cruise in Florida to the Bahamas for our family reunion. It was the first time I had been on a vacation where I didn't feel embarrassed or not want to participate in activities because of my body. It was the most freeing feeling.

I did everything that trip. Jeff and I went parasailing, then I went Snuba diving (yes, Snuba) with my daughter and nephew. We tried new things, I went in the water in my bathing suit and marveled at events that only people who have lost a significant amount of weight can appreciate: standard towels that wrap around my body, one size fits all robes, sliding into any booth without anxiety or fear. It was living.

Vacation or not I was still in marathon training mode. I made it a point to get up at 5am and run around the jog track on the boat. I often ran into several of my family members who were still awake from the night before! The trip was beautiful and relaxing. It was wonderful to see our family all together like that. Not everyone could go but those that did made is very memorable.

Not long after the cruise I went on a women's retreat with my church. When they first announced the retreat I was highly skeptical because I'm not into camping or communal living. I was told it wasn't tent camping but cabins so I should be fine. Clearly, these people don't know me.

I called the retreat center and asked if they had private accommodations. I was so happy to hear that they did. The following week at church they announced that we had cabins set aside for us. I would've felt like such a tool if I went with my group and then had my own quarters. The unrest I felt was surely the Holy Spirit. Sometimes not in words or even in whispers, just the feeling that you know what you should do. I was going to go with my group and get over myself.

We got to New Hampshire on a beautiful fall weekend in September. The leaves were already turning and the weather was crisp and perfect. I was sharing a room with five other women with a connecting door to 6 other women. This is definitely out of my comfort zone. I got to the cabin first and one bed was a double the rest were twin sized. I leaped on that double bed! It was also right by the door so I could slip out and run in the morning.

I always find the most peaceful and prayerful times is when I'm out in nature. From the moment I hit the hiking trails I knew that this experience was going to be something special. God was in every breeze through the trees and the morning fog on the lake. Yes, God is always everywhere but sometimes His presence is palpable. Almost tactile.

We had a lot of options for bible studies, group projects, boating, rifling, and speakers. We also had the option to spend some time alone. As much as I wanted to just solo this venture I know I was called to share my space with people.

I'm the unlikely introvert. Most people when they meet me think that I'm very social and fun – and I am – but I'm also a very introverted person. I value my alone time and after a while of social interaction I need silence and peace. My husband fully understands this about me. If I'm working on a project that requires a lot of "people time" as soon as I go home he's the first one to have a chai ready and is prepared for me to decompress for a while. It's a beautiful thing when people know you like that. Being on this retreat was definitely going to challenge that because there will be precious little time that I would actually be alone.

The first morning I woke up before dawn and went for my run. It was pretty dark so I stayed in the camp until the sun rose and then hit the trail. My reason for this was two-fold. The first was marathon training but I really didn't want to be in the room when everyone was waking and getting ready and taking showers. I timed it so when I returned most everyone was a breakfast and I could get ready alone. I was at the retreat sharing a room with a half a dozen people... I was sufficiently stretched.

One afternoon, I was going to listen to a speaker but the room was packed so I decided to get my bible and read by the water. I could've read it on my phone app but sometimes I need to feel the paper in my hands. I went into my cabin and one of the women was there. We got to talking because earlier that year she had a brain aneurysm and due to the keen eye of her daughter, the quick actions of the medical team, and the all mighty grace of God she walked out of the hospital with minor complications. That doesn't happen every day. I was like a reporter asking questions and she was so kind and open and answered everything. Throughout her recovery her daughter was sending updates to our prayer chain at church and we were praying for her health and well-being and here she was answering my questions just a few months later. I never knew just how important those questions would be to me just a few days later.

The retreat was amazing. Edifying in so many ways. I got to learn about the women in my church family on a whole new level, I met women from all over New England with stories to tell and things to share. I spent the weekend feeling the very tangible presence of God everywhere I turned. I returned home feeling refreshed, renewed, and ready to take my marathon training to the home stretch.

Thursday, September 22, started out as an unusual day. Jeff was working from home and I quit my job the previous month so we were both home all day. That never happens. The weather was beautiful and we decided to take the pups for a walk. Over Memorial Day weekend we solidified a new addition to our family, a 10 year old Chihuahua named Taxi Fitzgerald. We tried several times to get her to use a leash but the Her Royal Highness Queen of Everything Taxi Fitzgerald would hear none of it. We became the people we swore we would never be: the people who have a stroller for their dog.

On this beautiful, unseasonably warm September day we took our babies for a walk to the private beach. We got home and our beautiful day took a sudden turn.

My mother called and asked me to come over and she sounded concerned. She said that my sister was in a car accident and she didn't have any details she was heading to Massachusetts as soon as my Dad returned.

My dad drives for a ride sharing company and was completing a run and would hurry home when he dropped off his rider. We immediately went to my parent's house and waited for a few minutes before we realized we could take Mom and Dad could hop on the highway and meet us there.

We got to the hospital and my brother and my brother in law were already there. In the waiting area we learned that my sister's car accident was not the significant event that day. While she was in surgery with the trauma doctors they discovered that she had a brain aneurysm that ruptured while she was driving. The first doctor didn't have much for bedside manner and when we asked how serious her condition was she said that it's usually not survivable. I remember watching my mother crumble.

Suddenly, a peace washed over me. God filled my heart with this message: *They don't know. Only I know.* I told my parents and my siblings that only God knows what the future for my sister is and we need to leave it in His hands. For non-Christians the concept of leaving something entirely to God is difficult. We can knock on the throne room door and ask for anything but we must handle with grace whatever He deems the answer to be.

When the next nurse came in to speak with us I was armed with an arsenal of questions. My conversation at the retreat with my friend's mom who survived her aneurysm was playing back in my mind. I knew what to ask, what procedures could be done, and even more detailed questions about her recovery process. She looked at me with a confused look and asked if I worked in the medical field.

We waited and waited for an update on her progress during surgery. When I went to the cafeteria to get a drink I saw there was a little chapel across the hall. I walked in and I fell to my knees in front of the altar. I prayed like I have never prayed before. Before I was saved I used to pray for what I wanted or what I needed. It was always about me. Now I knew exactly what I needed to pray for in this circumstance. I needed to pray for God's will and my ability to handle whatever His will would be in this situation. If my sister was to be called home I only ask that I am able to help support my parents and my siblings through the pain and grief and I would need His help and the peace that only He can provide. It can be so easy to trust God when things are going well but the true test is to still trust and believe when you are faced with something that will rattle you to the core. I had to be ready for whatever may come and let my faith not waver in the circumstances.

We tend to think of things linearly. There's a beginning and an end. There's a start and a finish. We can't even begin to conceive that the God has no time. Everything is woven together and often we never know how one thing sets off a confluence of events that won't make sense until hundreds of years later. However, sometimes, we are blessed to see those events unfold immediately. Like a retreat that I really wanted to spend alone He compelled me to spend it with my church family. Then the speaker I wanted to hear was full so I went back to get my bible to read. I entered my room and saw my friend's mom who I never had a long conversation with before and ended up talking for nearly an hour about something 5 days later would be incredibly important. Even the nagging feeling at my job that compelled me to leave actually left me with time available to help my family care for my sister when we needed it most. God doesn't call the equipped, He equips the called.

As far as my sister I will only say this, she's recovering very well. God has blessed her tremendously. I never would've believed that totaling her car was the best thing to happen to her in that situation but it was. However, that is her story to tell and I hope that one day she shares it because it's amazing. If you ever questioned the existence of God you need to hear this story. I will continue to pray that she tells it.

The marathon was 45 days away and my running was suffering between trips to Boston and the emotional toll of not knowing how my sister's recovery would be or what it would take. When someone's in the hospital it's an all hands on deck situation for the entire immediate and extended family. Her husband and children were absolute warriors through this process and you really see love in action.

I wasn't even sure if I was going to be able to run in November. It seemed almost crazy to head to NYC not know what is happening from one day to the next.

My sister is a competitive person, college basketball coach, with drive for days. As she started to improve I asked her if she minded if I went to NYC for the marathon. She made it clear that she would be upset if I didn't go.

I was NYC bound.

CHAPTER SEVENTEEN
THE LONGEST MARATHON

We get to NYC and discover our hotel is above Hershey's Chocolate World. It's almost a cruel joke to put a formerly 400lb person in the same space as a world of chocolate. Looking over the city from the 19th floor of the corner room was amazing. The city is so beautiful in its own way. I'm definitely a country girl now but I will always remember my city roots.

The NYC Marathon is the largest in the world. There are nearly 70,000 runners! My friend who was going to run with me decided she couldn't make this year so I would be running alone.

Jeff and I head to the race expo to get my race bib and check in and it's overwhelming. There are so many people there but it was well organized. I found my bib in moments and there was a large wall with markers and you could write why you're running on it. I found a corner and wrote: I lost 250lbs to run! Jeff took my picture and a cameraman saw it and asked to take a picture of us. So incredible.

Our next stop was the pre-race dinner for the charity where we got to meet people and bond before the big day. It was a great event. We got to see the efforts of our fund raising and hear some incredible stories of survival and perseverance.

Although I missed all the long runs in the city one of the race coaches came to the podium and said this:

Don't forget the amount of effort that went into you being here. If you followed the training program then you ran 841 miles over these past few months. That's like running from this spot to Chicago, South Carolina, or Montreal.

He said that just as I was looking around the room getting more and more intimidated by the lack of body fat in the room and starting to question if I should be there. That question was certainly answered!

The next morning came very early. Breakfast was at 4:30am and we had to board the busses by 5:15am to make it to the race start on Staten Island. It was cold that morning and I had a long wait before I ran. My plan was to dress in layers and slowly remove what I no longer needed along the way. They had a ton of collection boxes all along the route for discarded run wear that gets cleaned and donated to the homeless.

My brother in law made t-shirts for my sister with a picture of her on the front and I knew that I was going to wear it. I needed to have her with me. She was definitely going to help me get through this challenge that was twenty years in the making. I dressed in layers but I had her close to me. When you wear a shirt with your name on it at the marathon spectators will cheer for you by name. My shirt said RAMONA STRONG on it and I wanted to hear her name with every step I took.

I was in the last wave with an 11am start. Getting to the start at 6am was woefully early and I decided to bundle up a lot. At the last minute I decided to wear thicker socks because it was really cold outside and I was going to be out there for a while. New York City closes the roads so everyone getting to the marathon had to get over to Staten Island as early as they could. Some went by bus, some by cab, and others by ferry.

Going over the Verrazano bridge from Brooklyn to Staten Island was so cool. It was sunrise over the Narrows and it was the last moment of peace. It's a view I'll never forget. Our bus was one of hundreds of busses approaching Starter's Village. I was glad I was alone because there was no pressure to stay with anyone or to lose anyone. The first thing I notice is that it felt like every nationality, every race, every age, every body shape and every language was represented here. The joy was overflowing. Several race teams had tents set up for the runners and I made my way to our tent. It was packed. I found a tiny unoccupied spot and sat down.

I can come across as very extroverted but I'm really quite shy especially in large crowds where I know no one. It was easy to look around and see that for many people marathons are a team sport. So many people were in groups that I started to question my love of being alone when training. A woman in her mid-twenties sat next to me and we exchanged friendly smiles.

One great benefit of being alone is that you disappear in a crowd especially when there are so many people in groups. I was able to sit and listen to the stories of camaraderie, training, fears, failures, missing toenails, and body chaffing and many more eventualities of marathon running.

There were four waves of runners and with each wave the number of people in Starter's Village started to decline. The first wave had the elite runners who can finish 26.2 miles in just over 2 hours. My brain still cannot conceive of running in a full out sprint for that long. Human bodies are amazing.

I was in that final fourth wave of runners. We consisted of charity runners, fast walkers, and people who will run about 13 minute miles or more. As the disembodied voice calls our wave to the start in ten different languages, Starter's Village finally looked empty after 4 hours of non-stop hustle and bustle.

Making my way to the corral I did another look around. My fears of being the largest runner at the marathon were quelled immediately. There were all types of shapes, sizes, physical capabilities, and reasons why everyone was toeing the line that day. I was one of a sea of people who had something to prove to no one but themselves. It was time.

I was in the last corral of the last wave and as I made my way to the start there were a line of portable toilets. If there's one thing that I cannot deal with its portable toilets. On this day, however, one thing I didn't want to deal with was holding my pee for nearly thirty miles. There were nearly 70,000 runners that day and about 65,000 have already passed through this area making my desire to use the portable toilets even less than before. I decide that it's better to do it now then on the course with no idea when the next round of toilets would be on the course. We were already notified several times that peeing on or over the bridge would have you removed from the race. I decided to risk it. I was surprised at how clean they were considering how many people have already been through this area.

I make my way back into the sea of people heading to the official start on the Verrazano Bridge. It was almost surreal going there. One of my favorite things was that each wave had a woman singing the National Anthem and a water cannon going off in the Narrows to start the race. I thought only the elite group would get that treatment. It was a nice touch.

I wasn't quite to the bridge when the cannon went off and people started running. The bridge has an upper and a lower deck and my corral was assigned to the lower deck. As I pass the official start I was struck by the beauty of New York City from the bridge. You can see Manhattan and soon enough we'd be running over there. Some people were stopping to take pictures and selfies but I didn't want to do that. I wanted to stay focused and finish strong.

The bridge from Staten Island to Brooklyn is two miles long and there are no spectators allowed on the bridge. Those first two miles was the quietest in the history of running. Lots of breathing, lots of intensity, a couple of selfies, but mostly people just beginning.

Just as my shirt told a story I saw a lot of stories out there. I ran next to a man who had a tag on the back of his shirt that said he was 80 years old and he was running is 40th NYC Marathon. He's run every single NYC Marathon since they started the 5 borough run! He's 80 years old and still running. That's how you start a marathon.

The first two miles went by quickly and

when you leave the bridge you take a left and then a right into a neighborhood in Brooklyn. That turn will forever be the closest I will ever feel to being Beyoncé in my life. As soon as you round the corner there were hordes of spectators holding signs, cheering loudly, and calling you by name. It was as far as the eye could see and I choked up a little. I was actually here. I was really doing it and hearing RAMONA STRONG with every step, just like I imagined!.

The signs were another highlight. People can be funny, creative, and downright insane with their signs. The first sign read:

Good job! There's only 24 miles to go!

I laughed a little then the thought tried to occupy my brain that I really do have 24 more miles to run. I couldn't let that thought take root. I can do this.

I was born in Brooklyn, NY, and we moved to Rhode Island before I was four years old. Most of my family still lives in New York and we spent a lot of time there over the years. Running the first leg of the marathon in Brooklyn, I saw so many familiar names. I was tempted to take my phone out and take pictures for my parents when I saw these places but I really couldn't afford to get side tracked.

One of my favorite things on the entire route was the churches. There were so many different denominations but each one had a musicians outside singing. From the choir of a Spanish Catholic Church to Baptist Gospel Choir down the road each church sang their praises to God in their own way while keeping Jesus at the forefront of my day.

Running after weight loss surgery has its own special circumstances. When everyone else is carbo-loading for long runs, I have to have a different approach since excessive carbs is no longer in the program. On my training runs it took a lot of trial and error and conversations with my nutritionist to get the right amount of fuel to get through longer runs. I learned this lesson the hard way one day when I missed the mile marker on a trail and ended up running out an additional two miles making my scheduled 14 mile trip up to 18 miles. I called my husband to let him know that I was struggling but I was going to try to press on. This was also in the height of the summer and the heat was oppressive. I made it to 15 miles and had him come and pick me up. After that lesson, I was always sure to add branch chain amino acid to my water and have some lite granola or packs of almond butter with me. The marathon was no different. I had low sugar craisins in one pocket, almond butter packs in another, and some granola for good measure.

At eighth mile I was doing well but I started to notice that my left foot was beginning to hurt. Although I thoroughly put runner's glide everywhere, I was developing a blister. It was also really warm. I had to focus and stay with it. I didn't want to focus on my foot but it was like when you accidently bite your lip and all you want to do it touch your lip with your tongue. All I could focus on was my foot. I was started to question if I'd be able to finish.

Next thing I see is the bus. The Struggle Bus. This is the bus the marathon puts out to pick up the injured, the tired, those that just can't complete the race. I thought back to my half marathon in 2008, when I was telling myself that if I just laid down the ambulance would bring me to the finish. I wasn't getting on that bus. Isaiah 40:31 was on repeat in my brain.

By the 10th mile I noticed that I wasn't feeling too well. I was hot, my foot hurt, and I wasn't even half way done yet. I needed to slow down and get some electrolytes in me.

186

Then I hear a voice yell, "Go GIN!" That is the nickname that my family has called me since I was a child. I turn around and there is my brother Richard with his daughter Ishanti and they have a sign cheering me on. I had no idea until that moment how much I needed to see them.

My big brother and niece stayed with me for 2 miles! I needed that support, I needed that love, I needed that sign and I never knew I needed it. At mile 12 there was an Aid Station. I sat for a minute, got some electrolytes, hugged my family, and continued on. I saw the Struggle Bus go by again but I wasn't getting on it.

At the half marathon marker I noticed that they were taking down the road barriers. The last wave runners were halfway through but they only keep the roads closed for so long. Those of us that take a little bit longer would have to finish the race with traffic on the roads and large markers removed. What I didn't realize is that those markers also had the tracking devices in them. It was at this time that anyone following my progress online lost me and had no idea where I was on the route, if I was hurt, or didn't finish. I didn't realize that for hours.

The pain in my foot was worsening as I crested mile 14. Less than a mile earlier I saw so many people both ahead of me and behind me yet I seem completely alone on the route. I double checked to make sure I was on the right path and I was but where did everyone go? I crossed a bridge from Brooklyn to Long Island City Queens so I knew I was still in the right place. For the first time, I was actually afraid. Maybe I'm not going to make it. God, please protect me out here and keep me on the path of this race.

"Hi, how are you?"

I never saw her before I heard her voice and she was right next to me. She was wearing her marathon race bib and literally appeared out of nowhere.

"I'm fine," I said. "My foot hurts but I'm hanging in there."

"You too? I have a horrible blister on my foot," she said.

We bonded right away sharing our blister war stories and how we both wore the wrong socks that morning. She lives in Brooklyn and runs the marathon almost every year with her running club. She ended up being the most helpful person to have on this run.

Things I didn't know:

- When they take down the markers they also take down the aid stations so no more water for the next 12 miles!

- You should bring a credit card if you'll need water or anything for the rest of the route

- If you buy something in a store they will let you use the bathroom so you don't have to use the portable toilets.

WHERE WAS SHE MY ENTIRE LIFE?

The best part of having a companion was that I was able to share this experience with someone. This was something that I never expected to enjoy.

Kathy was originally from the West Coast and moved to NYC in 2001, a few short months before September 11th. She was a trained clown at Ringling Bros. and had some incredible stories to tell. Listening to her made the miles go quickly and before you knew it we were out of Long Island City and in Manhattan.

In my training I thought I'd be done within 5-6 hours. Training on the bike path alone is very different from running with 70,000 in the streets of the city. My monster blister made that not a reality. We continued on sharing stories of our lives and making progress.

At mile 19 we were a little turned around. The aid stations and markers gone we had to rely on the map of the route. Since I struggle to find my way out of a wet paper bag, we had some issues getting around. There were still many racers on the roads and everyone has their own path they're taking. At one point we were with a man from Denmark and he was adamant we had to cross the street. We didn't think so. We ended up going our separate ways and he ultimately found us again. That's the beauty of the NYC grid system of streets. Eventually, you'll find your way. We found our way to mile 20 in The Bronx where there's a sign on the bridge that reads.

MILE 20 WELCOME TO THE WALL

I chuckled because I clearly hit the wall at mile 14. I was so happy to see mile 20 because

I trained on the South County Bike Path which is 7 miles. From mile 20 I just had to do one last trip of the Bike Path. I've done it so many times. I just have to pull through. Even at this point there are still spectators on the roadways cheering us along, making small talk, and encouraging us. There is no friendlier city than NYC on Marathon Sunday.

The last few miles were by far the hardest. I was exhausted, my feet were killing me, and my left foot was just about unbearable. I can do it. I can make it.

At mile 21 my husband called me and I was immediately concerned. Why would he be calling me? He was looking for me on the route because they lost track of me at mile 13 and he was freaking out. I had no idea that he was trying to text me. I had my phone on do not disturb but his call showed on my watch. I asked him to go to the finish line because I would really need him at the finish line. I didn't want to see him before because if I stop I don't think I'd be able to start again. He said he'd meet me at the finish.

The cobblestones of Fifth Avenue are beautiful and I've always loved them. Running over them with blisters changed my appreciation of them a bit. Kathy and I entered Central Park for mile 24 and we were nearly finished. I've been to Central Park plenty of times yet I never once noticed how hilly it was. As we crest one hill and start the way down I remember thinking that it's just as painful going down the hill as going up. This will be the longest 2 miles of my life.

The like a rocket something goes flying by us. I see a man in a wheelchair flying down the hill and I thought for sure he was going to spill out! Two race guides are running past us to catch up to him.

We end up catching him making our way up the next hill. He gains a lot of ground on the downhills but to make it up a hill he has limited use of his feet and arms.

"Hi!" he says with exuberance.

"Hello! How are you? Is this your first marathon?" I ask him.

He starts to laugh. His guide tells us that this is his tenth marathon. For ten straight years this man has gone 26.2 miles in NYC in a wheelchair with limited use of his legs and hands. On the straightaways he uses his feet to move his chair. It can be a very slow process so he makes up for it with his fearlessness on the downhills. I was in awe of him. We heard his laugh cascade loudly down the next hill. It was like fuel to keep moving for me.

As we make our way to the end of Central Park we see a woman with a baby carriage and she screams "Oh my goodness! You're Ramona Strong!"

I look at her quizzically because I wasn't sure if she was reading my shirt or if she knew me.

"I've have spent the past hour with your husband. He is so proud of you." She hands me bottled water and paper towels.

"My husband is here?" WHY IS HE NOT AT THE FINISH LINE I'm thinking.

"He's not that far. What a sweetheart. And you, oh my goodness, you've overcome so much! And your sister, just know we are all praying for her recovery."

"Thank you so much. I'm sorry I'd love to stop and properly thank you but I can't."

"I understand! You're almost done and close that husband of yours. So happy for you!" she yells and disappears around a corner.

Just as I was telling Kathy that I wanted my husband at the finish line because my entire body hurts, I don't want to stop, if I see him I'm going to stop, and then I won't finish, and I'm so close... There he was standing at the mile 25 marker like an ethereal vision. I was instantly so happy that he didn't listen to me at all. I hug him while jogging in place and tell him I love him but I can't stop. He tells me he loves me and he'll see me at the finish. It was so fast I thought for a second that maybe I was hallucinating. We pressed on.

The last mile was crazy. I was rounding out my marathon experience and thinking back to the days when walking was a chore. I thought back to the many times I dreamed of doing this over the years when it seemed so impossible. I remembered the first walk I took with my daughter and it was over before it started. Later I discovered I went 200 steps. I thought of how running was always something I needed to do alone but here I was with someone and I was never so happy to have her with me.

As we approach the finish they have flags set up for every single country represented in the race. It's almost overwhelming to be there. To see it from this perspective. We are both battered and blistered and tired but we decide that we are going to make sure we run it all the way in.

We get to the finish line, hands raised in victory, and there's a race official who hugs us and crosses with us. I see my husband and the officials let him place my finisher's medal over my head. Tears are flowing from my face as I hug Jeff hard. Every ounce of my body hurts.

I look over and I see Kathy and I hug her and we are both crying because we did it. We really dug deep and finished it.

"Thank you so much," I tell her. "I don't think I could've done this without you."

"Thank me? If it weren't for you I would've hopped on the subway and went back to Brooklyn hours ago!"

I hugged her like I knew her my entire life. I meant every ounce of feeling and emotion in that hug. At the start of the race I wondered if I missed something by being alone and by the end of the race it was confirmed. There's a joy and comradery in running long distances that I needed to embrace. I never saw Kathy on the race route before that moment in Long Island City when God sent her to me to keep us both accountable and motivated. If you want to truly get to know someone, spend 12 miles in pain together.

I get back to Jeff and I'm wrapped in my baked potato covering heat retaining blanket from the marathon aids. I grab my post-race swag bag and I'm ready to limp back to the hotel and crash. I look at my watch and I've gone over 66,000 steps and 33 miles! The miles kept adding up from getting to the start, walking around starters village, and finally to the actual start of the race.

"Jeff, where's the car?" I asked through tears, pain, and emotion.

"I walked here," he responded.

I tried not to pass out immediately. We were about 15 blocks from the hotel but I know that after the last 33 miles that was not going to happen. We walked toward 5th Avenue and a Pedi cab comes by! Jeff flags him down and we venture back to the hotel.

I'm still in my baked potato wrapping, holding Jeff's hand, looking around the city as our driver pedals through crazy NYC traffic. I'm trying to ignore the pain in my feet to soak in this moment. The breeze on my face and profound sense of accomplishment in my heart. I spent so many years of my life running away from feelings and problems that it was overwhelming that I set out to do something so far beyond my scope of ability just a few short years ago.

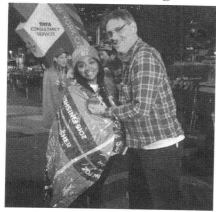

Surrender. It was all in the surrender. When I first accepted Christ I had to surrender. I lived for so long in my own strength, made decisions out of fear, and was paralyzed by my anxieties. It found it very freeing to place those things in His hands. It wasn't until my 42nd birthday that I finally surrendered my weight to Him. It was from that moment that every barrier was opened to me. I was able to release the feelings of guilt and shame that food had over me. I was able to find my strength in HIS strength and that made all the difference.

I can do all things through Christ who strengthens me. Philippians 4:13 NIV

Which was a good thing because I had to call upon all of His strength to get me out of the Pedi cab and into the hotel.

I sat on the edge of the bed and stared at my feet. I was afraid to take shoes off because my feet hurt so badly that I didn't want to see what they looked like. I decided to take my right shoe off first since that one had just regular running pain where my left foot felt like it was on fire. My right shoe came off just fine but when I took my sock off I was met with a bit of a surprise. I had a blister on the top of my big toe that was bigger than a quarter and the size of a jawbreaker! That is the foot that doesn't hurt! I gingerly took off my left shoe and then my left sock. I was expecting missing toenails, bruising, or something equally horrendous to look at and my foot looked fine. I tilt my foot to look at the bottom and I see what was causing all the pain. I had a blister underneath a large callous across the center of my entire foot. It was the size of a credit card and it was super tender to touch. The next few days were going to be interesting to say the least.

After the half marathon, I learned the importance of moving and stretching immediately after finishing. I wasn't going to attempt to make it to the fitness center with my feet the way they were so I decided to do some stretches on the bed. I had to loosen up or I'd stiffen up. After a few minutes of stretches I tiptoed to the beautiful bath that Jeff drew. I spent the next hour soaking and letting everyone know I made it.

In the tub I kept my eyes on the NYC Marathon Instagram page and just saw miracle after miracle cross the finish line. At my half marathon I was really dead last and I thought for sure I would be here too. Not even close. Until the wee hours of the morning they were still crossing the finish line. There was a woman who did all 26.2 miles with one leg on crutches. It took her nearly 13 hours to complete but she did it. I even saw the man I saw back in the corral talking to his friend about why he wanted to do the marathon. He said he was 400lbs and he hadn't done anything for so long that he wanted to prove to himself that he could do it. He did it. I felt his story in the depth of my person. I completely understood.

Ninety minutes after completing the most arduous challenge of my life this lifelong insomniac fell asleep without incident for the first time in years.

CHAPTER EIGHTEEN
THE FIVE F WORDS

I spent most of my life fighting my body. I hated it. I hated every roll, every flab, every ounce of subcutaneous fat that seemed to be all over my body. My identity was also completely tied to my weight. I was fat. I remember seeing a meme on Facebook one day that really changed how I approached my identity in my weight.

You're not fat, you have fat.
You also have fingernails.
You are not fingernails.

After reading that the first of many epiphanies happened with the way I saw myself and my weight. I always considered

201

myself as fat. I AM FAT. That reads like fat is the very essence of who I am and that's exactly what I considered myself. But when you take the same concept and apply it to fingernails you see how unbelievably ridiculous it is to view yourself that way. After that day I was no longer fat! I happen to have fat but that fat doesn't change the core of who I am, the essence of my being, or my place in the world.

I've tried so many diets, so many quick fixes, so many expensive treatments and nothing ever worked. After surgery I noticed some pretty incredible things about myself that really changed my approach to weight loss and wellness.

Many people will say that if post-surgical dieting is so much work then why couldn't you do it before surgery? This is a valid question. What I can say about my personal experience is that the surgery allowed my body to take a break so my mind could catch up. Long term weight loss success is a mental game as much as a physical one. In the past, when the mental game became too hard I would easily quit and revert back to past behaviors. Surgery removed that option. I had to learn how to live and challenge myself to learn how to live WELL after weight loss surgery. That became an art form that I credit to the **Five F Words of Weight Loss**.

1. **FAITH** – As I mentioned throughout this book that in my past I always considered my weight MY problem. It was my personal issue that I held in a tightly closed fist. Even after I came to a saving knowledge of Jesus Christ, I still held on to my weight even after I was able to let other issues go. Weight was mine. After fully surrendering my weight on my 42nd birthday, I noticed the first major change in the way I handled my weight. It was no longer mine. Like my anxiety and fears I was able to hand my weight to the Lord and no longer hold it. It was the realization that not everything that weighs you down is yours to carry. I had to let Him carry it and He always wanted to! The tenant of Let Go and Let God applies to weight loss. Aside from removing that burden from your shoulders, a firm foundation in faith also gives you a place of refuge that you will need when things get tough. I'm not joking when I tell you that on many occasions it was only by the grace of God that I didn't

dive into a vat of ice cream! I pray daily for the strength to continue on this path, the ability to show His grace to others with their weight issues, and protect me from cravings which can be debilitating some days! Faith is the very first necessary step in my weight loss.

2. **FAMILY** – I believe the goals of long term weight wellness is to be able to eat as a family. This will require understanding and support. If you have a family like mine then you may be thinking that you need to have the support of your entire large family. Technically, you don't have to have the support of anyone to be successful – it just makes it a lot easier if those influential people in your household are on board with what you are doing and are willing to help you along the way. Influential people are the adults living in your household, spouse, partner, parents. Influential people in your household are not children (hold on, don't freak out). Children take their cues from adults and although change isn't easy for many people children will adapt to your lifestyle. Sitting down and dining

together is one of the best ways for
families to come together and
communicate. In these busy times, it's
all but lost, but in those moments when
you do have the privilege of dining with
your family the last thing you want is to
prepare separate meals for everyone. If
you have surgery, then after the required
time that you are on pureed foods you
should really try to make something for
the entire family. It took a clever
amount of time to prove to my husband
that we could both eat and be satisfied.

There's also the issue of the inner circle
and outer circle of family and
acquaintances. Weight loss by any
means is a personal and emotional thing.
Some people tell everyone about their
methods of losing weight and others tell
no one. That is entirely up to you as an
individual. Share what you want or share
nothing based on your comfort level. I
decided to share openly for two reasons.
The first is that I am a notorious closet
eater who is completely untrustworthy
with food and I needed the
accountability of people knowing what I
was doing with permission to call me

out if things looked a little out of whack. The second reason was I wanted to talk to someone real – not on the internet – about weight loss surgery. I had questions and there was so much junk on the internet it was hard to sift through what was real, what was opinion, and what was straight garbage. That openness was my choice. Please note that with that choice comes some issues. You will open yourself up to all types of scrutiny from people who do not understand the process of weight loss surgery, the lifesaving benefits of weight loss surgery, or how it's not the quick fix easy out that people seem to think. Steel yourself to it. The thoughts of your inner circle matter; those adults in your life that have influence over you and your living situation. I would strongly advise that you not concern yourself with the opinions of any other people.

3. **FOOD** – I know this seems a bit obvious, but food is definitely a factor in weight loss but in many ways. For years food was the answer to any

question I ever had. Now, if hungry isn't the question food is never the answer! Food is wonderful and when prepared well is very tasty but ultimately, food is a fuel source. Before I eat I have to do my Ten Second Rule. That's where I take 10 seconds and ask myself a few questions: Am I hungry? Is this on plan? Will eating this keep me on track for my goals? Is it nutritious? If it passes those questions then it's safe to eat. For a person who spent years eating mindlessly this was a very difficult thing to   master.

Here's another thing about food. This was one of the most critical changes in my understanding of wellness and weight loss success. For years I considered my body a punishment and dieting was the awful thing that I did to make my hideous body less hideous. The critical change occurred when I decided to love my body instead of hate it. When you love something it's easier to take care of and nurture. I wanted my body – my amazing temple from God – to function well and move with ease. In order for that to happen then I had to be conscious of what I was putting in my body. I thought of all the things I wanted to change with my body over the years. I hated my arms. They were large and jiggly and I would never, ever show my arms. I would wear sweaters at the beach so as not to show my arms. Then I realized that these jiggly arms hugged my grandfather before he died. I thought of the rubbing and chaffing and embarrassment of my thighs. I would blow out the crotch of my pants so often from the rubbing and chaffing. I hated it so much. Then I realized that in all my hatred of the rubbing and chaffing with every step I took I failed to realize and be grateful for the fact that I was walking! How could I not see that? My body had value, it had beauty, and it had worth before I ever lost a pound. Now, I strive to show that love of my body with every bite of food, with every step I take, with every word I speak about my body it will reflect the love with which it was created.

4. **FITNESS** – Another seemingly obvious thing that would be integral to long term weight loss and wellness.

Movement is essential to living. Humans are spending more and more time sitting and becoming more sedentary. The impact to our health is obvious. The catchphrase is *Sitting Is The New Smoking*. Let that sink in! Picture any major city filled with high rise office buildings and at any given there are thousands of men and women sitting in office chairs with curved spines typing on keyboards with various ailments. Carpal tunnel, lumbar and cervical spine issues, low back pain, herniated discs, obesity, dehydration, and poor nutrition. Not only is what we eat important but how we move and how often we move can help ward off a lot of the issues we see these days. You don't have to run a marathon to improve your fitness levels. Start small. Make a goal to touch your toes and work a few minutes each day and track how long it takes you accomplish that task. Small, incremental goals will lead to success but be sure to have the same outlook as with food: workout because you love your body not because you hate it. If you miss a day, be gentle with yourself and remember another day is another opportunity to get it right. One bad day doesn't ruin progress, it just delays it a little. You can rebound. God's mercies are new each day. I think of that often because it's so true and would think of how many times I just bailed on something when one day didn't go my way. I should've recognized the setback and continued forward but I never could do that. I would get angry an just forget it all. The art of being gentle with me was a slow process but so valuable.

5. **FEELINGS** – I ate my feelings all the time. I ate my problems and my insecurities too. What happens when you no longer have food as a coping mechanism? For me, I had to learn how to handle disappointments, fears, and anger without resorting to food. This required me to be able to safely and effectively find and use my voice. I've always been a better writer than in person communicator. I find that when I write I can get manage my thoughts and not worry about my emotions coloring what I'm trying to say. When I try to speak in person - especially about

something sensitive or that I'm passionate about – I could let my emotions get the better of me and then I lose my words or my point entirely. I had to learn to speak my feelings, be honest with myself and others since I would normally just say that nothing was wrong when something was really wrong because I didn't want to discuss it. I'd stew over it and down pints of ice cream and let it go that way. That was no longer going to be an option. This was one of the hardest things for me. Thirty years of habit is not easily broken.

This was also the F word that ties all of the others together. In dealing with my feelings I had to call heavily upon my faith, learn how to eat food without being ruled by my feelings, I had to learn how to communicate issues with my family expressing my feelings, and sometimes I'd hit the gym and sweat out my feelings.

Joshua Rosenthal said that "wellness isn't a destination, it's the vehicle." I loved this quote because it opened a new perspective on wellness for me. For decades, I was looking for a place of health, but it isn't a place at all. I wanted to arrive at a healthy place with a healthy weight. Yet, it isn't a place at all! In the same vein, I never cared for the term "weight loss journey" because I felt that I was already on a journey of life and weight loss is a part of that larger journey. Combining those two thoughts is how I came up with my blog title Navigating Weight Loss. My journey was already well in play before I took on the challenge to improve my wellbeing, but what I vehicle I was in for the journey needed attention. I spent many years on a raft trying to paddle with my hands across the ocean but as time passed and my knowledge and effort grew I was able to trade in my raft for a kayak, then a rowboat. With each passing day and new lesson learned, I am improving with a goal of arriving to heaven when He calls me with my mind and spirit properly reflecting the love He has shown.

This process is a winding road of discovery. Discovering who I am without food. Discovering how to handle emotions without food. Discovering what my body can do without food. Discovering if I can be strong enough to avoid food. Discovering that you can never truly be without food, so you discover that it's really this:

Discovering who I am
without **focusing** on food.

Discovering how to handle emotions
without **using** food.

Discovering what my body can do
without **abusing** food.

Discovering how all the strength I need comes from Jesus! Every day I strive to keep Him first and life becomes less about food and more about Him.

And for all of this I am grateful.

FINAL WORD

"Comparison is the thief of joy."
Teddy Roosevelt

I hope this book sheds a little light on my personal experience dealing with weight and navigating the emotional and physical work of weight loss. There is one thing that I feel is important to note, this is just one person's story and every person will have their own unique experience. No two weight loss stories are the same so your story may be different from mine.

I remember my first post op support group and I had lost 100 lbs in just a few months. There was a woman next to me who lost 45lbs in a longer amount of time and she was visibly upset at the differences in our weight loss. She allowed my weight to dull her shine. Losing any amount of weight when you are working so hard for it requires celebration and should never be influenced by another person's results. Be honest with yourself and gentle with yourself through this process and with faith you can do it.

God Bless,

Regina

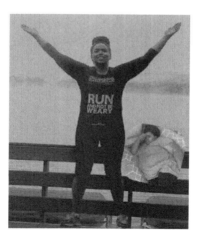

ABOUT THE AUTHOR

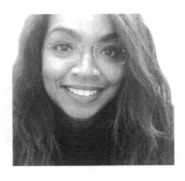 Regina Bartlett is a blogger and speaker from the gorgeous Rhode Island coastline where she spends her days with her amazing husband Jeff and their combined family of six adult children and two very tiny adorable Chihuahuas. Her first book, *Healthy Fare: Bariatric Friendly Recipes and Helpful Guides* can be found on Amazon. She's active in her church, sings on the praise team, and is amazed every single day at how God has totally changed her life. After completing her marathon goal, she set her sights on another childhood dream: becoming a Black Belt in Shorin Ryu Karate. You can read about her adventures in life on her blog at reginabartlett.com.

TL;DR: Wife, mother, writer, avid crafter, lover of Jesus and tiny dogs everywhere with a story to tell.

Made in the USA
Middletown, DE
14 April 2018